Mommypedia

DR. AMRITA SAHA

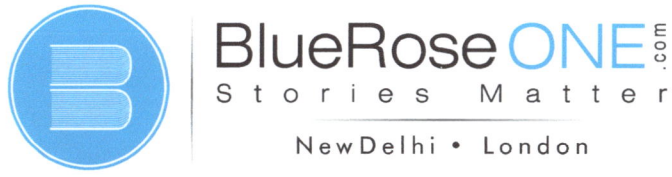

BLUEROSE PUBLISHERS
India | U.K.

Copyright © Dr Amrita Saha 2024

All rights reserved by author. No part of this publication may be reproduced, stored in a retrieval system or transmitted in any form or by any means, electronic, mechanical, photocopying, recording or otherwise, without the prior permission of the author. Although every precaution has been taken to verify the accuracy of the information contained herein, the publisher assume no responsibility for any errors or omissions. No liability is assumed for damages that may result from the use of information contained within.

BlueRose Publishers takes no responsibility for any damages, losses, or liabilities that may arise from the use or misuse of the information, products, or services provided in this publication.

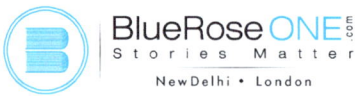

For permissions requests or inquiries regarding this publication, please contact:

BLUEROSE PUBLISHERS
www.BlueRoseONE.com
info@bluerosepublishers.com
+91 8882 898 898
+4407342408967

ISBN: 978-93-5819-594-1

Cover design: Tahira
Typesetting: Tanya Raj Upadhyay

First Edition: January 2024

Foreword: A Journey into the World of Mommypedia

Dear Readers,

Today, it is my utmost pleasure to introduce you to a remarkable guidebook cum scrapbook, aptly named Mommypedia. As I stand here before you, as a teacher and an admirer of the author's work, I am filled with an indescribable sense of awe and admiration for the passion, dedication, and expertise that have gone into crafting this invaluable resource.

I had the opportunity of witnessing tremendous improvements in the lives of both pregnant women and the medical professionals who advise them during my work as an instructor and mentor to aspiring gynaecologists. A gynaecologist's relationship with their patient is holy, founded on trust, compassion, and a shared commitment to nourishing life. Mommypedia emerges from this sacred space, a testament to the countless lives touched and transformed by the author's expertise and unwavering care. This book, dear readers, is far more than a mere compilation of medical knowledge and advice. It is a beautifully curated scrapbook, capturing the essence of the awe-inspiring journey of pregnancy. Within its pages lie not only the scientifically precise guidance that every mother-to-be craves but also the gentle reassurances and heartfelt wisdom that make this book a true treasure.

As I delve into the intricacies of Mommypedia, I am struck by the author's ability to strike a delicate balance between the clinical precision of a seasoned gynaecologist and the empathetic understanding of a trusted confidant. The chapters unfold seamlessly, guiding expectant mothers through the myriad of physical, emotional, and psychological changes they may experience during this transformative period. From the wonders of conception to the nurturing care of the developing fetus, this book illuminates every step of the miraculous journey, providing support and solace to mothers and their loved ones.

Mommypedia is a testament to the author's passion for empowering women and ensuring the well-being of both mother and child. The author's deep-rooted commitment to education and care shines through each meticulously crafted page. The inclusion of interactive elements, anecdotes, and practical tips transforms this guidebook into a compassionate companion, comforting and guiding expectant mothers through the unpredictable twists and turns of pregnancy.

With heartfelt sincerity, I encourage all readers, whether expectant mothers, fathers-to-be, or healthcare professionals, to embrace Mommypedia as an indispensable guide in navigating the beautiful yet often challenging journey of pregnancy. I firmly believe that the pages of this book will become a trusted ally, dispelling doubts, and instilling confidence in the face of the unknown.

To the author, I extend my deepest gratitude for sharing your expertise, wisdom, and compassionate nature through this remarkable work. Your dedication to the field of gynaecology and your unwavering commitment to nurturing life is an inspiration to us all. Mommypedia is an embodiment of your teachings, a legacy that will undoubtedly leave an indelible mark on the lives of countless mothers and their precious children.

May Mommypedia serve as a beacon of knowledge, guidance, and solace, illuminating the path of expectant mothers as they embark on the extraordinary journey of motherhood.

Sincerely,

T.S. Bag
Professor Department of Obstetrics & Gynaecology
Medical College, Kolkata

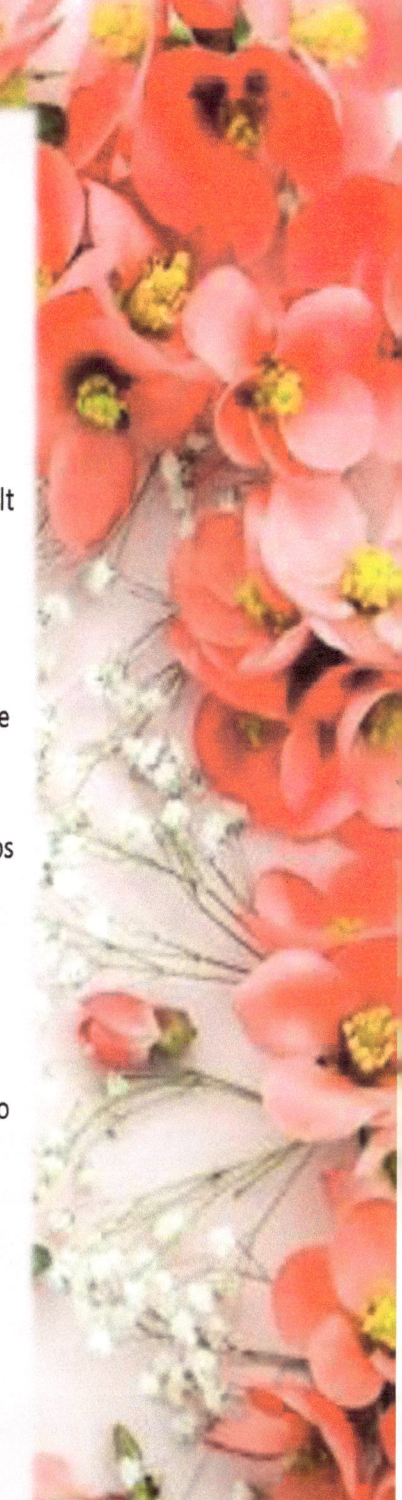

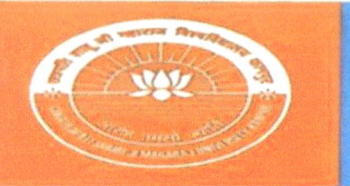

Chhatrapati Shahu Ji Maharaj University, Kanpur - 208024
(Formerly Kanpur University, Kanpur)

Prof. Vinay Kumar Pathak
Vice Chancellor

07 July, 2023

Foreward

The journey of pregnancy is a remarkable and transformative experience that brings joy, anticipation and sense of wonder. It is a time when a new life takes shape within and a profound connection is forced between a mother and her unborn child. Throughout her pregnancy a lady faces multitude of physical and emotional challenges

In this book, "MOMMYPEDIA" a scrapbook-cum- guide for pregnant ladies the author Dr. Amrita Saha has embarked on a captivating exploration of the various aspects of prenatal care, illuminating the knowledge, guidance and support that are integral to promoting a healthy and positive pregnancy experiences. Way beyond just the medical intervention and routine checkups, this books delves into a rich tapestry of topics providing a holistic prospective on the care required during each face of pregnancy and covers the emotional physical and psychological well being of a pregnant lady in holistic yet lucid manner.

I congratulate Dr. Amrita Saha, a renowned gynecologist of Kanpur city, for writing this book. I wish this book all the success.

(Prof. Vinay Kumar Pathak)
Vice Chancellor

कार्यालय/Office : +91-512-2581280
फैक्स/Fax : +91-512-2581280
ई.मेल/E-mail : vcocsjmu@gmail.com
वेबसाईट/Website : www.csjmu.ac.in

ACKNOWLEDGEMENTS

I am immensely grateful to the following individuals and entities who have played a significant role in the creation of this guidebook cum scrapbook, titled "Mommypedia: A Weekly Journey through Pregnancy."

First and foremost, I would like to express my deepest gratitude to my husband, Dr Ganesh Shanker whose unwavering support and encouragement have allowed me the freedom to pursue my passion and dedicate myself to this project. Your love and understanding have been instrumental in making this book a reality.

To my child, Abhigyan Shanker thank you for being an exceptionally understanding and self sufficient child and bringing immeasurable joy and inspiration into my life. Your presence has added depth to my understanding of motherhood, and it is because of you that I embarked on this endeavor.

I am grateful to all my teachers and my seniors in NORTH BENGAL MEDICAL COLLEGE AND MEDICAL COLLEGE KOLKATA for your patience and dedication in teaching me the art and science of Gynaecology & Obstetrics and for challenging me to push beyond my limitations. It is a testament to the invaluable impact teachers can have and without your mentorship, this book would not have been possible.

I would like to extend my heartfelt appreciation to my assistant Ms Anushka Awasthi, who worked tirelessly to design and bring this book to life. Your creative vision and dedication have made this project visually captivating and user-friendly. Without your invaluable contributions, this book would not have been possible.

A sincere thanks to Mr Akshay Sharma for giving the whole story a life from my scribbled script.

A special mention goes to my pg dr Monica Monpara, HOD, colleagues and senior residents in GMC Kannauj, the fellow gynaecologists and seniors in Kanpur Obstetrical and Gynaecological Society and physicians who have provided valuable insights and suggestions. Your expertise and guidance have enriched the content of this book, ensuring its accuracy and relevance.

I would also like to thank my patients, the women who have entrusted me with their care and allowed me to be a part of their journey through pregnancy. Your experiences and stories have served as the foundation for this book, and it is with deep gratitude that I acknowledge your contributions. You continue to inspire me every day.

To my parents, who instilled in me a love for learning and a drive for excellence, thank you for nurturing my dreams and supporting me throughout my career. Your unwavering belief in me has been my constant motivation.

Lastly, I would like to express my gratitude to God for blessing me with the opportunity to serve and care for pregnant women. Your guidance and grace have been my guiding light, and I am humbled by the privilege to be a part of such a transformative and profound experience in a woman's life.

To all those whose names may not be mentioned but have contributed in countless ways, I extend my sincere appreciation. Your support, encouragement, and belief in me have been invaluable.

This book, "Mommypedia," is a tribute to the beauty and significance of pregnancy, and it is my hope that it will serve as a companion and source of inspiration for all the expectant mothers who read it.

With heartfelt gratitude,

AMRITA SAHA

PREFACE OF BOOK

As a gynaecologist and obstetrician, as a gynaecologist I have joined this wisdom over years of my clinical practice that life of a woman in full of significant life event. Each such life eveny for potential to change the thinking and behavioural pattern of lade for rest of her days. Pregnancy, especially the first pregnancy is crucial times she needs support of family, friends, doctor everyone. But the person who's support she needs most is of "Her own MIND"

I have witnessed the journey of countless mothers bringing new life into this world. It is an incredible experience that brings with it a range of emotion and challenges that cannot be understated. I have been blessed to touch upon their lives by the skills God has bestowed upon me. It is for every stage of their pregnancy from the very first day

This boothe reason that I am thrilled to launch this book, which is designed to guide mothers throughout k is much more than just a guide; it is a scrapbook that allows mothers to document their thoughts, feelings and memories throughout their pregnancy. With colourful backgrounds for every section, mothers can capture every precious moment that they share with their little ones as they grow inside of their wombs.

In addition, the book is packed with useful articles on everything from postpartum care and diet to tips on taking care of one's body and mental health. It is my hope that this book will serve as an indispensable resource for all mothers, providing them with the guidance, support and information they need to navigate the wonderful journey of pregnancy.

Thank you for choosing to embark on this incredible journey with me, and I wish you all the very best for the incredible adventure ahead.

DEDICATION

To the expectant souls who have shared their fears and dreams with me, Whose vulnerability has fueled my passion to provide guidance, Thank you for allowing me to be a part of your remarkable journey.

You are embodiment of strength and grace.

May the words within these pages be a guiding light, Illuminating your path with wisdom, knowledge, and love.

May it serve as a companion throughout your miraculous journey, A treasure trove of memories for you to cherish.

With boundless admiration and gratitude,

    Dr. Amrita Saha [Gynaecologist and Author]

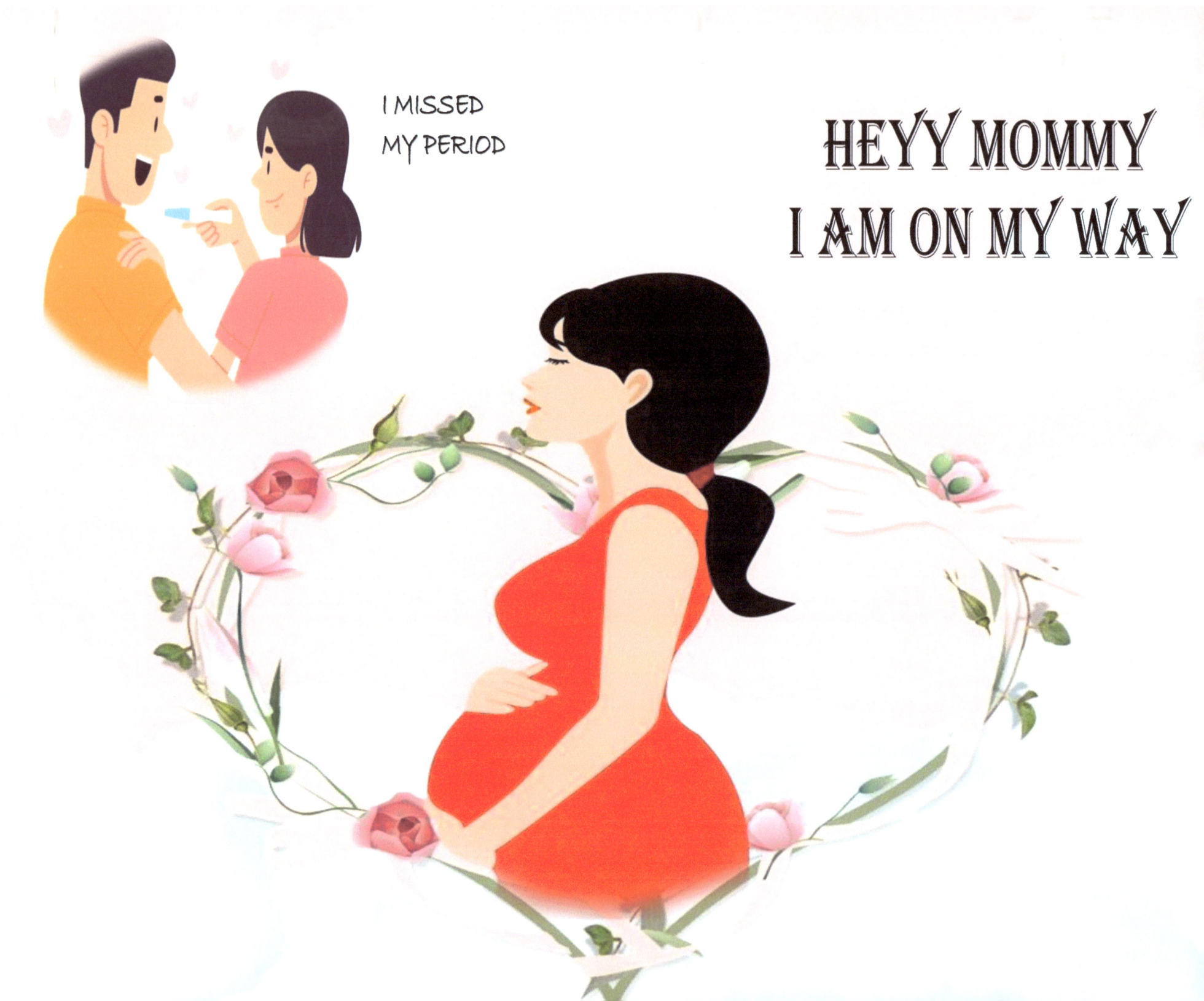

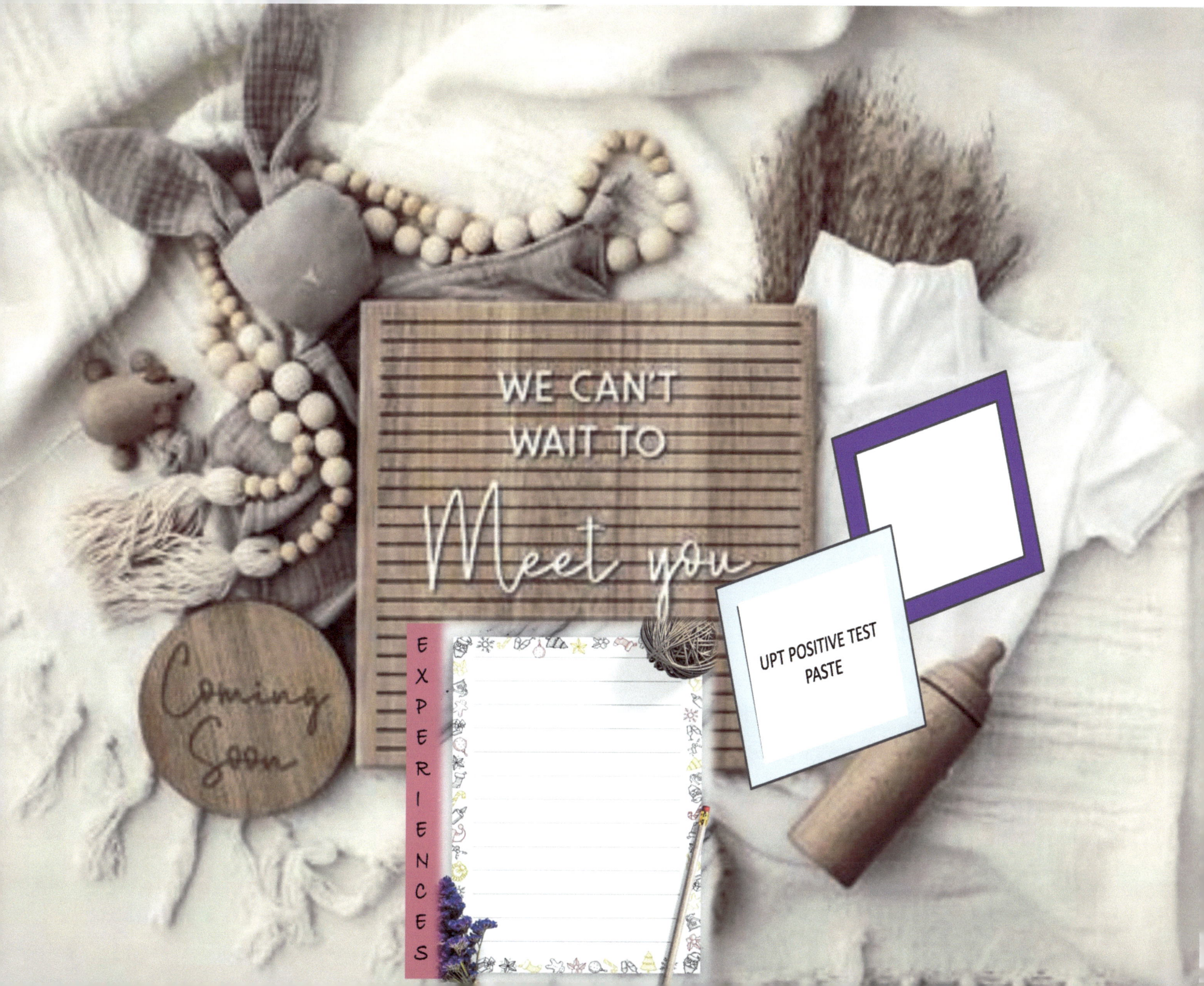

CHECK-UPS AND INVESTIGATION

The schedule of antenatal check-ups and vaccinations may vary depending on the healthcare provider and the specific needs of the pregnant woman. However, a general guideline for antenatal check-ups is as follows:

1. First trimester (weeks 1-12): Initial antenatal visit, usually within the first 6-10 weeks of pregnancy. This visit includes a complete medical history, physical examination, blood tests, and ultrasound to confirm the pregnancy and estimate the due date, NT NB scan and Dual Marker

2. Second trimester (weeks 13-28): Regular check-ups every 4-6 weeks to monitor the progress of the pregnancy. During this period, additional tests such as fetal anomaly scans may be conducted to check for any abnormalities in the baby's development. And specialized tests like Quadraple Marker and/or NIPT according to your Gynaecologists opinion

3. Third trimester (weeks 29-40+): More frequent check-ups every 2-4 weeks to monitor the well-being of both the mother and the baby. In the later weeks, check-ups may become more frequent, typically every week.

ANTENATAL VACCINATIONS

Antenatal vaccinations during pregnancy mainly include:

1. INFLUENZA VACCINE: Recommended during flu season to protect the pregnant woman and the baby from influenza-related complications.

2. TDAP VACCINE: Given between weeks 27 and 36 to protect against tetanus, diphtheria, and pertussis (whooping cough). This vaccine also provides passive immunity to the newborn baby.

3. Other vaccinations, such as hepatitis B, may be recommended depending on the woman's medical history, risk factors, and regional guidelines. It is important for pregnant women to consult with their healthcare provider for a personalized antenatal care schedule and to receive the necessary vaccinations for a healthy pregnancy.

PRECONCEPTIONAL

The role of preconceptional counselling is to provide information, support, and guidance to individuals or couples who are planning to have a baby or become pregnant. It aims to identify and address any potential risk factors or issues that may affect the health of the future child or the pregnancy itself.

During preconceptional counselling, various factors are discussed, including medical history, lifestyle choices, genetic conditions, reproductive health, and the importance of prenatal care. It may also involve recommendations for lifestyle modifications, such as improving nutrition, quitting smoking, managing chronic conditions, and addressing any potential environmental or occupational hazards.

COUNSELLING

PRECONCEPTIONAL

The goal of preconceptional counselling is to optimize the chances of a healthy pregnancy and reduce the risk of complications or birth defects. It can help individuals or couples make informed decisions about pregnancy planning, genetic testing, and prenatal care.

Prenatal genetic diagnosis, sometimes referred to as prenatal genetic testing or screening, involves assessing the genetic health and potential risks of a fetus during pregnancy. It is typically offered to individuals or couples who may have an increased risk of having a baby with a genetic disorder or who have certain concerns regarding their baby's health.

COUNSELLING

PRECONCEPTIONAL COUNSELLING

Prenatal genetic diagnosis can help identify genetic conditions or chromosomal abnormalities, such as Down syndrome or cystic fibrosis, before birth. It allows parents to make informed decisions about their pregnancy and, in some cases, to plan for any necessary medical or support interventions that may be required after birth.

It is recommended that individuals or couples who have a family history of genetic disorders, who belong to certain ethnic or racial groups with higher risks of genetic conditions, or who have previously had a child with a genetic disorder undergo preconceptional counseling and consider prenatal genetic diagnosis. Additionally, women who are older (usually over 35 years) may also be advised to undergo genetic testing or screening during pregnancy due to the increased risk of chromosomal abnormalities.

HAIR CARE IN PREGNANCY

General Tips

Stay Hydrated: Drink plenty of water to keep yourself and your hair hydrated from within.

Protect from Sun and Heat: Shield your hair from excessive sun exposure and limit your time in extreme heat. Wearing a hat or using a UV protectant spray can help prevent damage.

Avoid Chemical Treatments: Refrain from using harsh chemical treatments like hair dyes, bleaches, or perms, especially in poorly ventilated areas. If you wish to color your hair, consult with your healthcare provider or a professional stylist about safe options.

Remember, every pregnancy is unique, and it's important to consult with your healthcare provider before trying any new hair care products or treatments. They can provide personalized advice based on your specific circumstances.

HAIR CARE IN PREGNANCY

During pregnancy, hormonal changes can also affect your hair. While some women experience thicker and more lustrous hair, others may face challenges like excessive hair loss or changes in texture. Here are some hair care tips for each trimester of pregnancy:

FIRST TRIMESTER

Gentle Cleansing: Use a mild, sulfate-free shampoo and conditioner to clean your hair without stripping away natural oils. Avoid harsh chemicals or treatments that can potentially be absorbed into your bloodstream.

Scalp Care: Keep your scalp clean and healthy by gently massaging it while shampooing. This can help stimulate blood circulation and promote hair growth.

Balanced Diet: Ensure you have a well-balanced diet rich in vitamins and minerals, as they play a crucial role in maintaining healthy hair. Include foods like fruits, vegetables, lean proteins, and whole grains.

DIET CHART
NORMAL

$$BMI = Body\ weight/ Height\ (meter)^2$$

(BMI 18.5-23), 2260KCAL

MEAL TIMING	MENU AND AMOUNT
MORNING (6:30 A.M-7 AM)	NORMAL/LUKE WARM WATER (250 ML) MILK 200 ML + SUGAR 5 G (TSP) OR JAGGERY 10 G.
BREAKFAST (8:00 A.M)	DOSA (2) (RAWA)/IDLI (3)/ PARATHA (2) + GREEN VEG (50GM)/POHA (250GM)/ BOILED EDD (2) UPMA (200GM)/CHILLA (2) (75GM)
MID-MORNING (10:30 A.M)	SEASONAL FRUIT (1 ANY MEDIUM SIZE) (100GM). NO FRUIT CHAT
LUNCH (12:30-1:00 P.M)	RICE (2 KATORI 200 GM) OR ROTI (4) KATORI (CHICKEN/MEAT/FISH) OR 75 GM GREEN VEG
EVENING SNACK (4:00 P.M)	SEASONAL FRUIT (100 GM)/ NUTS (1/4 CUP OR 1 FISTFUL)
DINNER (8:00 p.m)	2 KATORI RICE/3 BAJRA ROTI KATORI DAL + 75 GM GREEN VEG
BED TIME (10 P.M)	MILK (200 ML) + 5 GM SUGAR

UNDERNOURISHED (BMI <18.5), 2410KCAL

MEAL TIMING	MENU AND AMOUNT
MORNING (6:30-7 AM)	NORMAL/LUKE WARM WATER (250 ML) MILK 250 ML + SUGAR 5 G (TSP) OR JAGGERY 10 G.
BREAKFAST (8:00 A.M)	DOSA (2) OR IDLI (3)/ PARATHA (2) +VEG (50GM) OR POHA (200GM)/BOILED EDD (2)/BREAD (2) OMELLATE (2) + UPMA (200GM)/CHILLA (2)
MID-MORNING (10:30 A.M)	SEASONAL FRUIT (150GM) NO FRUIT CHAT
LUNCH (12:30-1:00 P.M)	RICE (200 GM) OR ROTI (5) + 1 KATORI (CHICKEN/MEAT/FISH) OR 100 GM GREEN VEG + 1 KATORI CURD/RAITA + 75 GM SALAD
EVENING SNACK	(4:00 P.M) SEASONAL FRUIT (100 GM) + NUTS (75 GM OR 1 FISTFUL)
DINNER (8:00 p.m)	200 GM RICE OR 3 ROTI + 1 KATORI DAL + 90 GM GREEN VEG.
BED TIME (10 P.M)	MILK (200 ML) + 5 GM SUGAR

OVERWEIGHT

(BMI > 23), 21200KCAL

MEAL TIMING	MENU AND AMOUNT
MORNING 6:30 A.M-7 AM	NORMAL/LUKE WARM WATER (250 ML) MILK 200 ML (WITHOUT SUGAR OR JAGGERY).
BREAKFAST (8:00 A.M)	DOSA (2) OR IDLI (3)/ PARATHA (2) +VEG (50GM) OR POHA (1/2 KATORI)/ BOILED EDD (1) + UPMA (200GM)/CHILLA (2) (70GM)
MID-MORNING (10:30 A.M)	SEASONAL FRUIT (100GM). NO FRUIT CHAT
LUNCH (12:30-1:00 P.M)	RICE (90 GM) OR ROTI (3) + 30 GM (CHICKEN/MEAT) OR 30 GM + 1 KATORI CURD/ RAITA + 50 GM SALAD
EVENING SNACK (4:00 P.M)	1 CUP GREEN TEA + 1-2 BISCUIT/NUTS (1 FISTFUL)
DINNER (8:00 p.m)	1 KATORI RICE OR 3 ROTI + 1 KATORI DAL + 50 GM GREEN VEG.
BED TIME (10 P.M)	MILK (100 ML) (WITHOUT SUGAR)

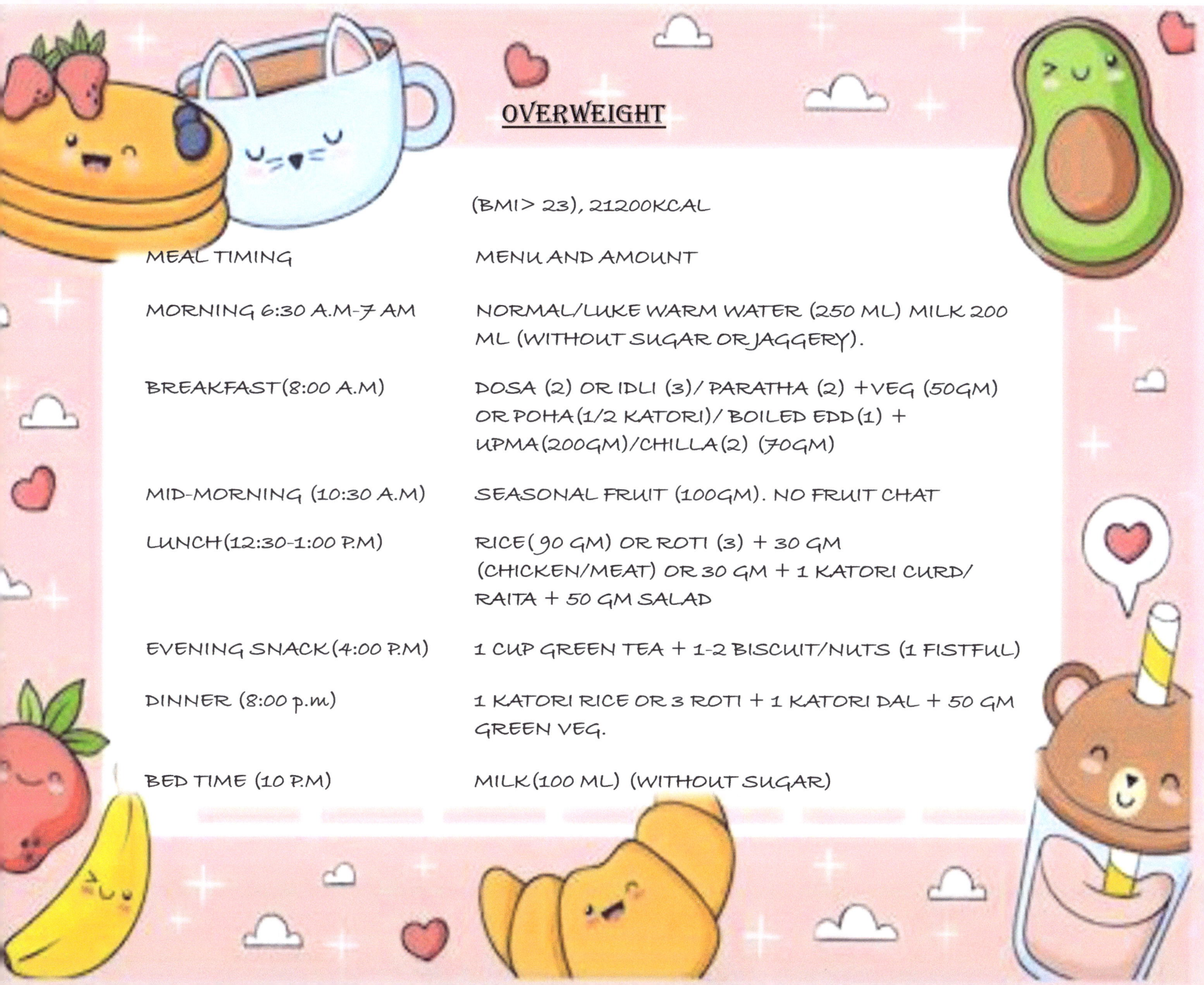

WEEK 4

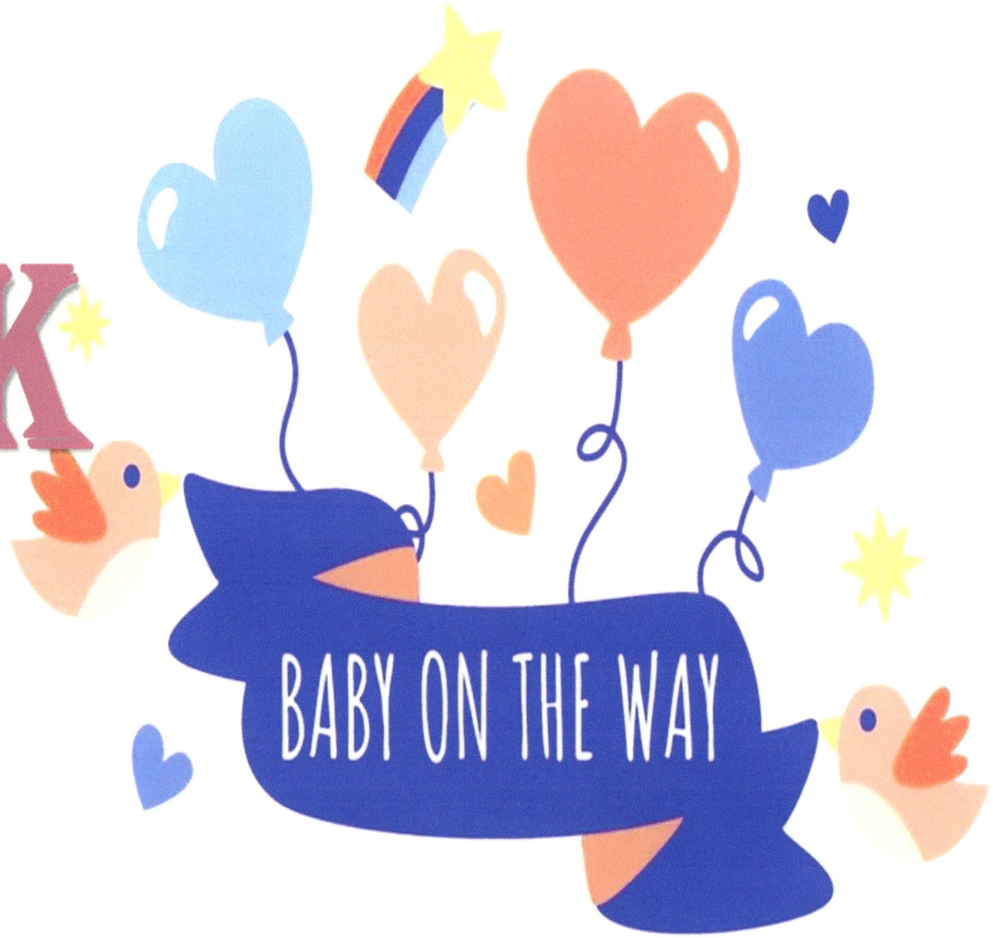

BABY ON THE WAY

LOWER ABDOMINAL PRESSURE

- Don't worry a feeling of pressure in your tummy or even mild cramping without bleeding is very common. Especially in first pregnancies, and is usually a sign that everything is going right, not that something's wrong.

- If bleeding is very minimal and for 1-2 days it's normal, but if it is more like period, consult a doctor. Don't take any counter medicines like analgesics painkiller without consultation.

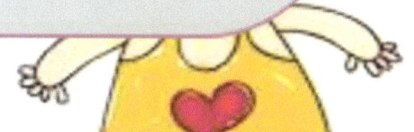

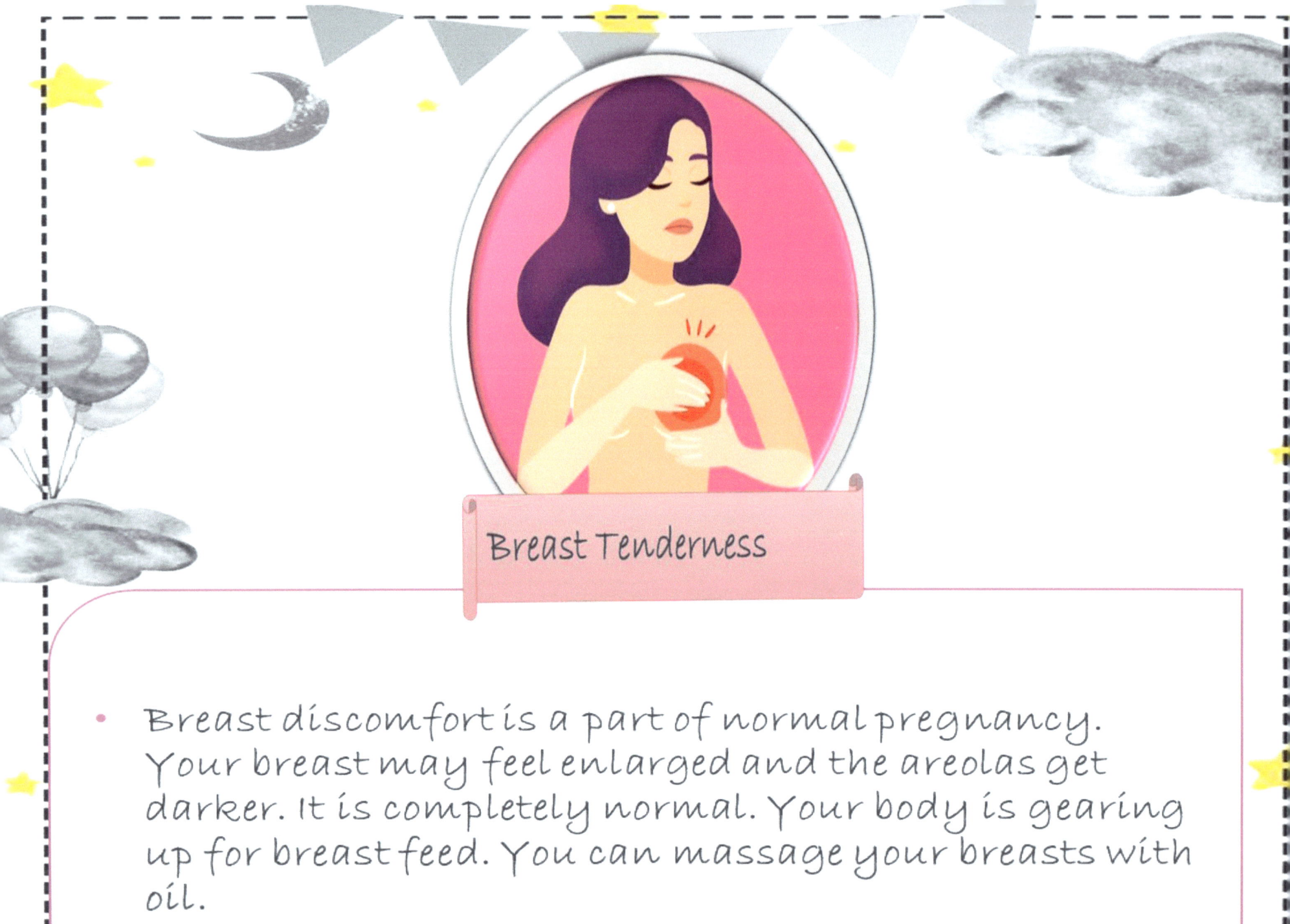

Breast Tenderness

- Breast discomfort is a part of normal pregnancy. Your breast may feel enlarged and the areolas get darker. It is completely normal. Your body is gearing up for breast feed. You can massage your breasts with oil.

SKIN CARE IN PREGNANCY

General Tips

Stay Hydrated: Drink plenty of water throughout the day to keep your skin hydrated from within.

Maintain a Healthy Diet: Eating a balanced diet rich in fruits, vegetables, and essential fatty acids can contribute to healthy skin.

Get Adequate Sleep: Sufficient rest helps rejuvenate your skin and promote a healthy complexion.

Remember, it's crucial to consult with your healthcare provider or dermatologist before introducing any new skincare products or treatments during pregnancy, as individual circumstances may vary.

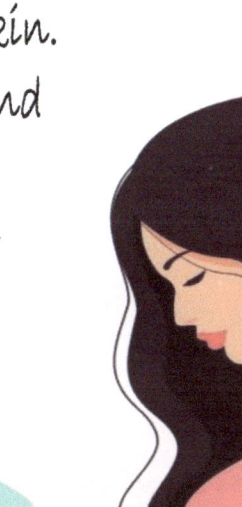

SKIN CARE IN PREGNANCY

First Trimester

Gentle Cleansing: Cleanse your face with a mild, soap-free cleanser to remove dirt and excess oil without stripping away natural moisture.

Moisturize: Use a gentle, pregnancy-safe moisturizer to keep your skin hydrated and reduce dryness or itching.

Sun Protection: Apply a broad-spectrum sunscreen with an SPF of 30 or higher to protect your skin from harmful UV rays. Look for products that are free from chemical sunscreens like oxybenzone or avobenzone.

Acne Management: If you experience pregnancy-related acne, consult with your healthcare provider before using any acne-fighting ingredients. Some over-the-counter options like benzoyl peroxide and salicylic acid may be safe in limited concentrations, but it's best to seek professional advice.

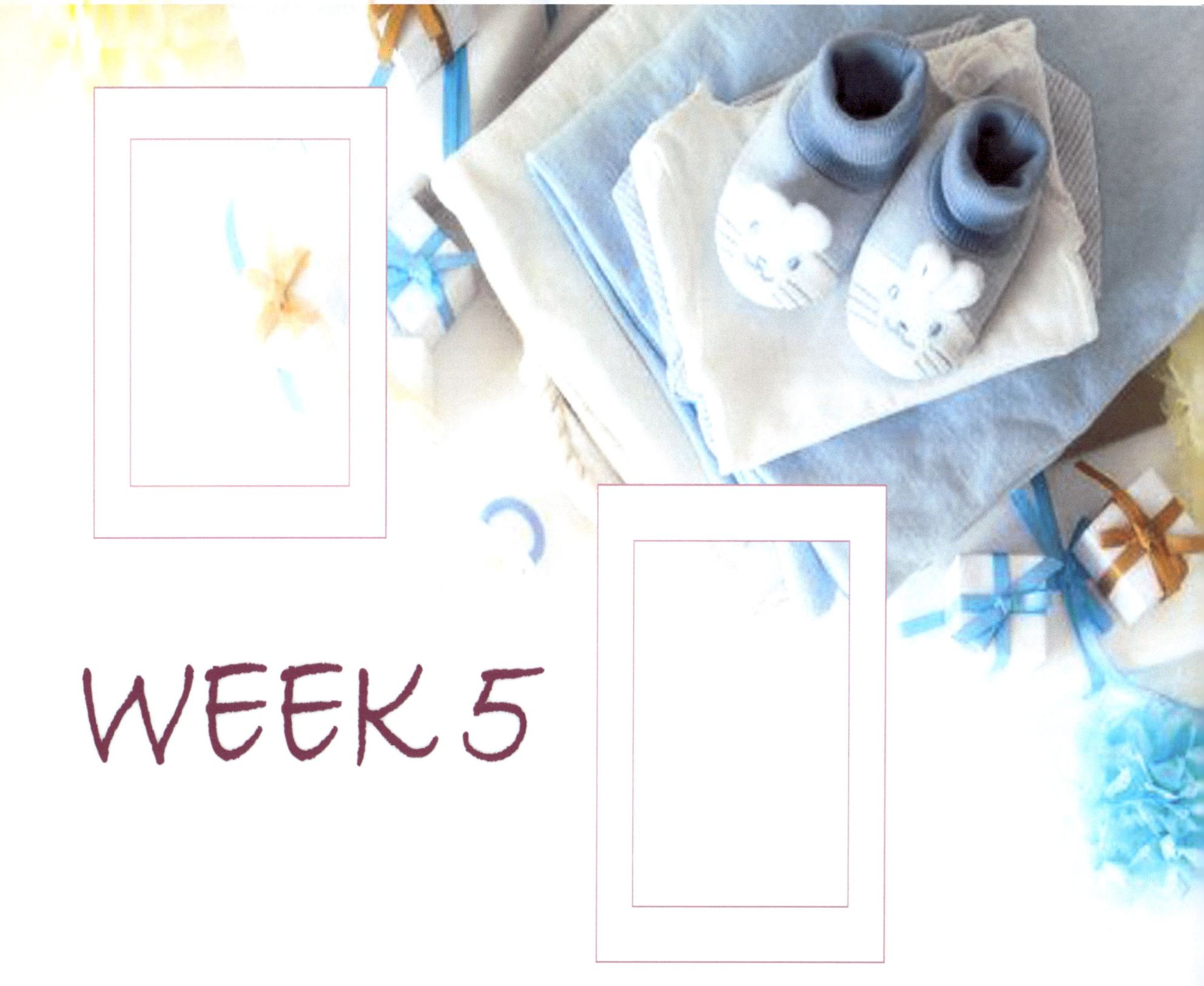

WEEK 5

EXERCISE IN PREGNANCY

Engaging in regular exercise and yoga during pregnancy can provide numerous benefits, including improved mood, increased energy, enhanced strength and flexibility, and better overall well-being. However, it's important to consult with your healthcare provider before starting any exercise routine, as individual circumstances may vary. Here's a general guide for weekwise exercise during pregnancy:

Weeks 5-12

During the early stages of pregnancy, focus on maintaining your current exercise routine if you were physically active before pregnancy. If you're new to exercise, start with low-impact activities such as walking, swimming, or prenatal yoga. Avoid activities that involve a high risk of falling or impact to the abdomen.

NAUSEA & VOMITING

It is very common in first few weeks, its time to get your comfort food

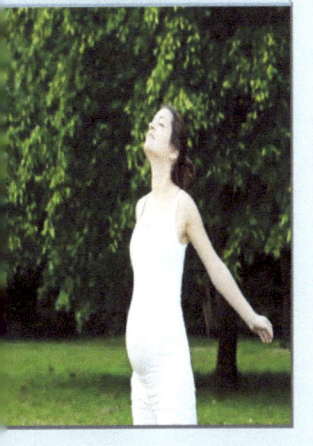

breath fresh air.

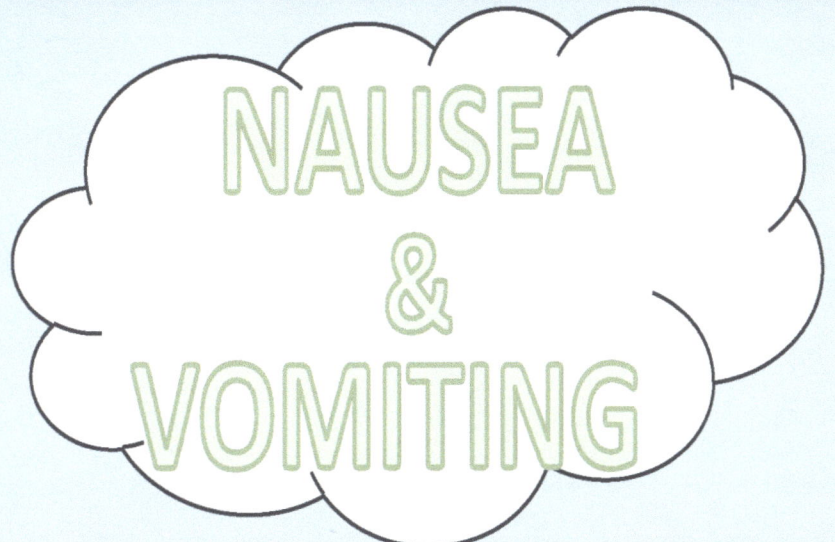

Always stay in a good ventilated surrounding.

Eat whole grain biscuits or a dry toast in the morning.

Eat smaller but frequent meals.

Drink plenty of fluids - Try Warm ginger honey lemon water also sip of water in between the meals.

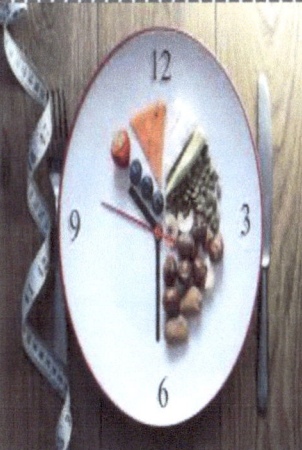

Don't skip meals- even if you don't feel like eating.

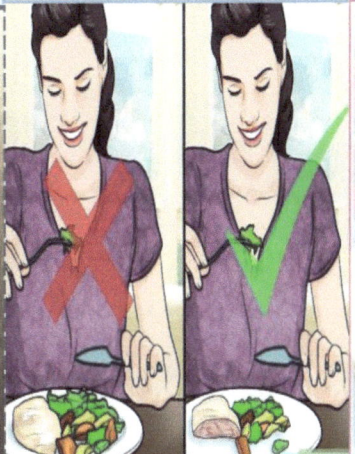

Try Dahi, watermelon, pasta, bananas, and berries. (Blend food is easy to digest).

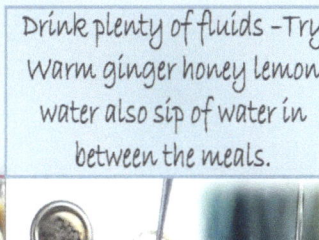

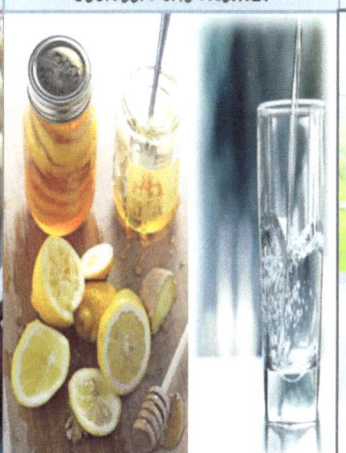

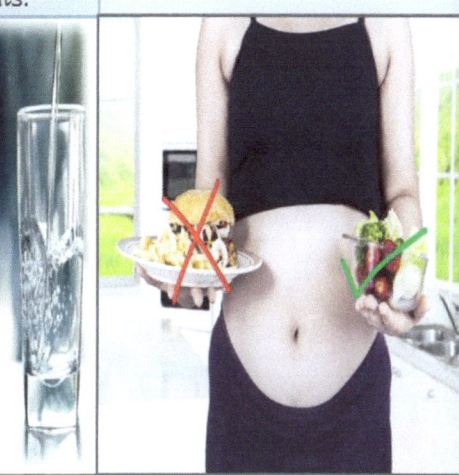

Don't eat greasy and spicy foods.

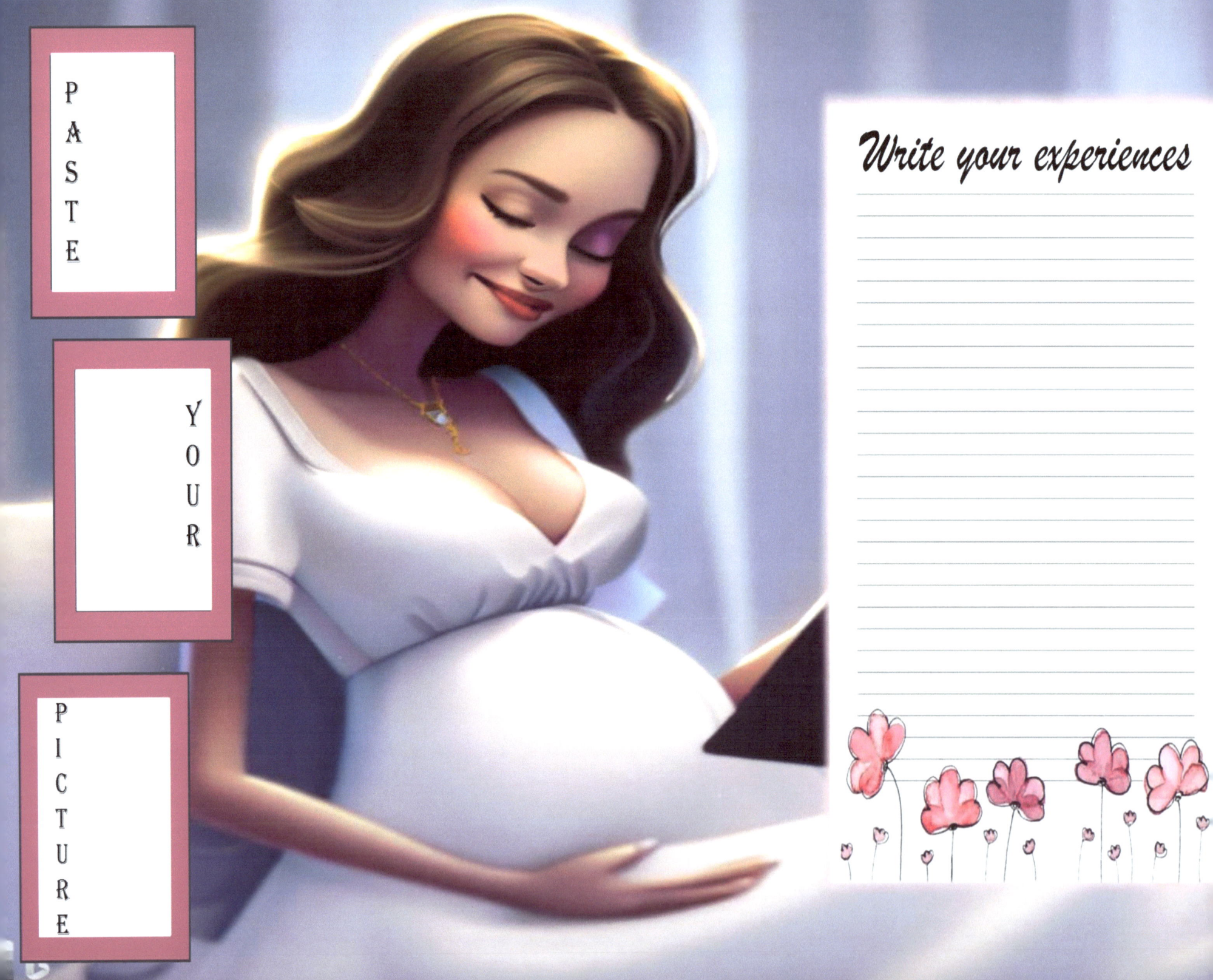

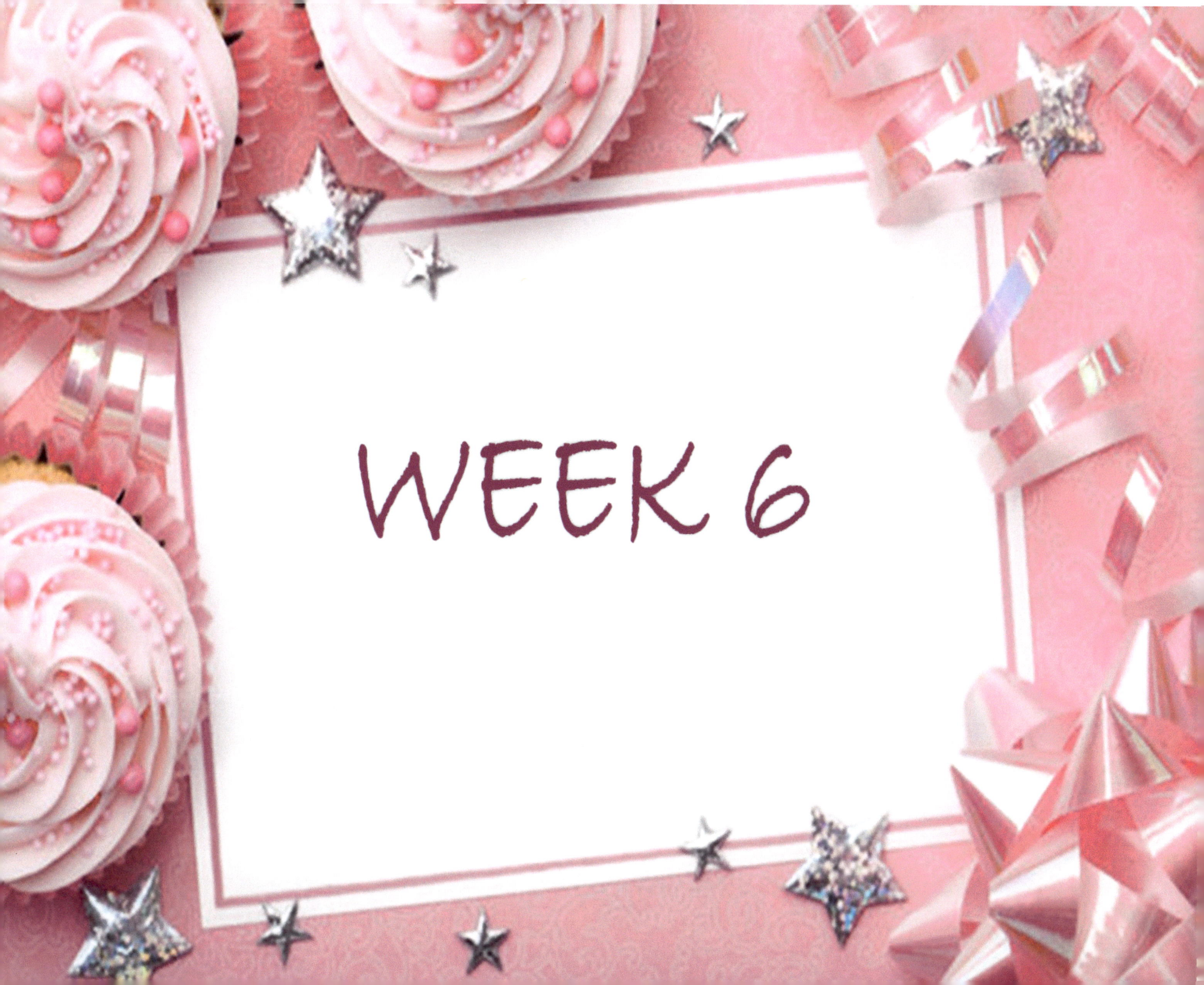

CURING CONSTIPATION

- Constipation is an all too common first trimester pregnancy symptom

- You must avoid foods that'll clog stomach, like refined white bread, Maida biscuits, processed or packed foods.

- Eating fibers: add whole grains, pulses, seasonal vegetables and fresh fruit in daily menu. Take enough water with plenty of fluids, particularly unsweetened.

- Finally remember that getting moving can keep things moving, another good reason to put exercise on the agenda. Ask your doctor about what kind of exercises you can opt for during these days.

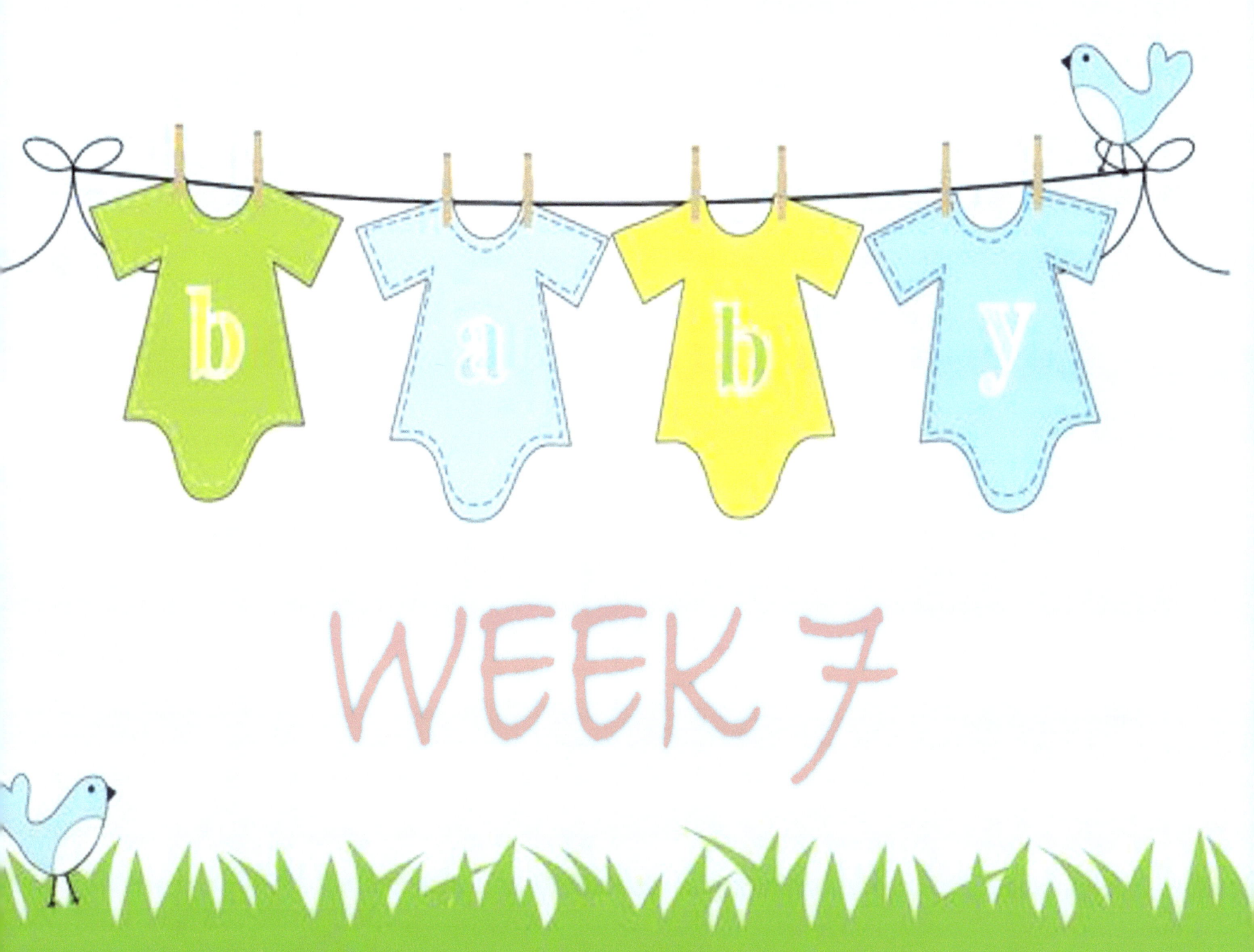

FREQUENT URINATION

- Frequent urination and need to pee a lot often starts in this early pregnancy and sometimes continues until the baby is born

- If you find you need to get up in the night to pee, try cutting out drinks in the late evening.

- However, make sure you drink plenty of non-alcoholic, caffeine-free drinks during the day to stay hydrated.

- If you have any pain while peeing or you pass any blood in your pee, you may have a urine infection, which will need treatment.

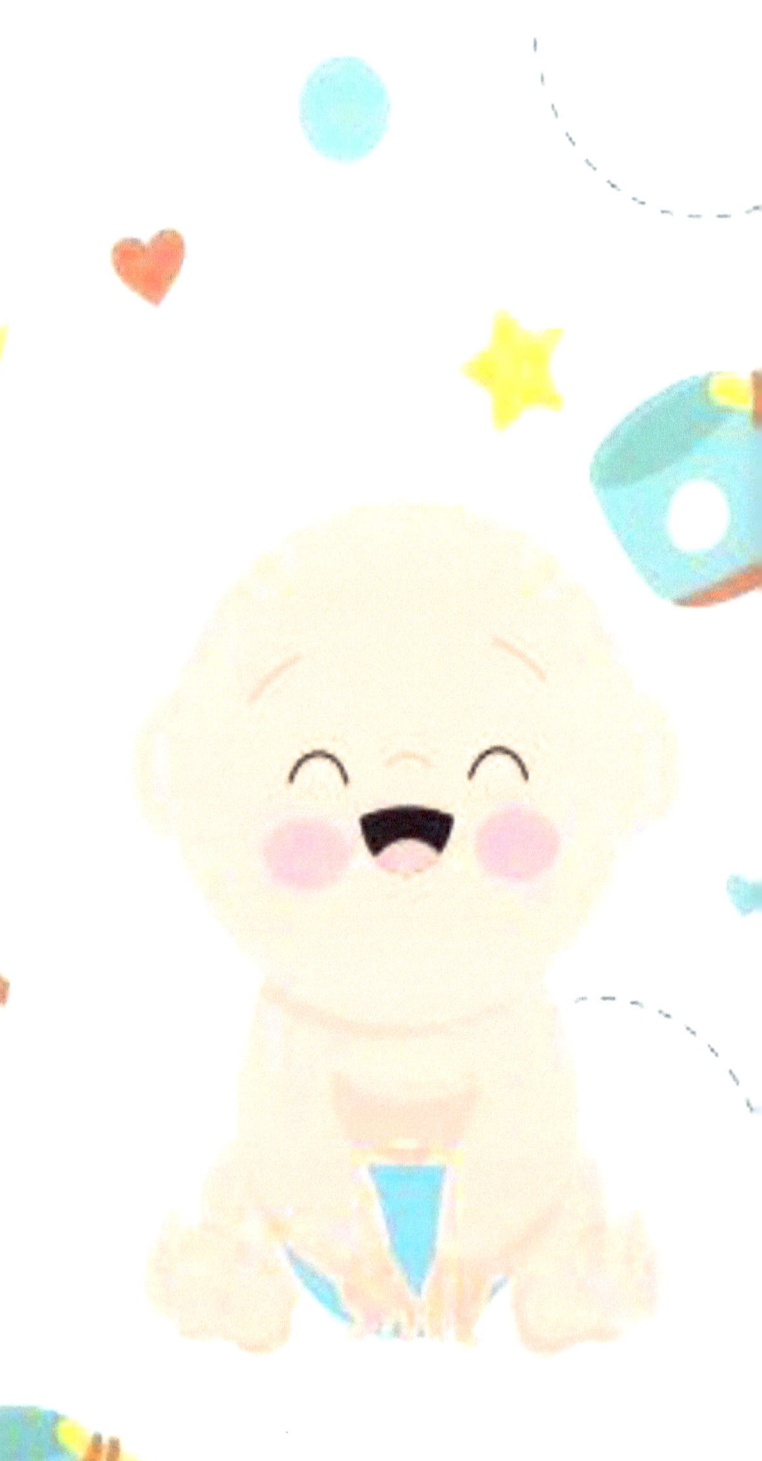

PASTE YOUR PICTURE

Write your experiences

before you are in

our arms

WEEK 8

Paste your photo

Paste your photo

you are in our

hearts

INCREASED VAGINAL DISCHARGE

- An increase in the estrogen hormone causes high blood flow to the area below the stomach, causes changes in the body's mucous membranes. This causes increase in the vaginal discharge.

- This discharge protects the birth canal from infection by maintaining a healthy balance of bacteria, so don't over clean it. Do not use any chemicals over the counter without asking your care giver.

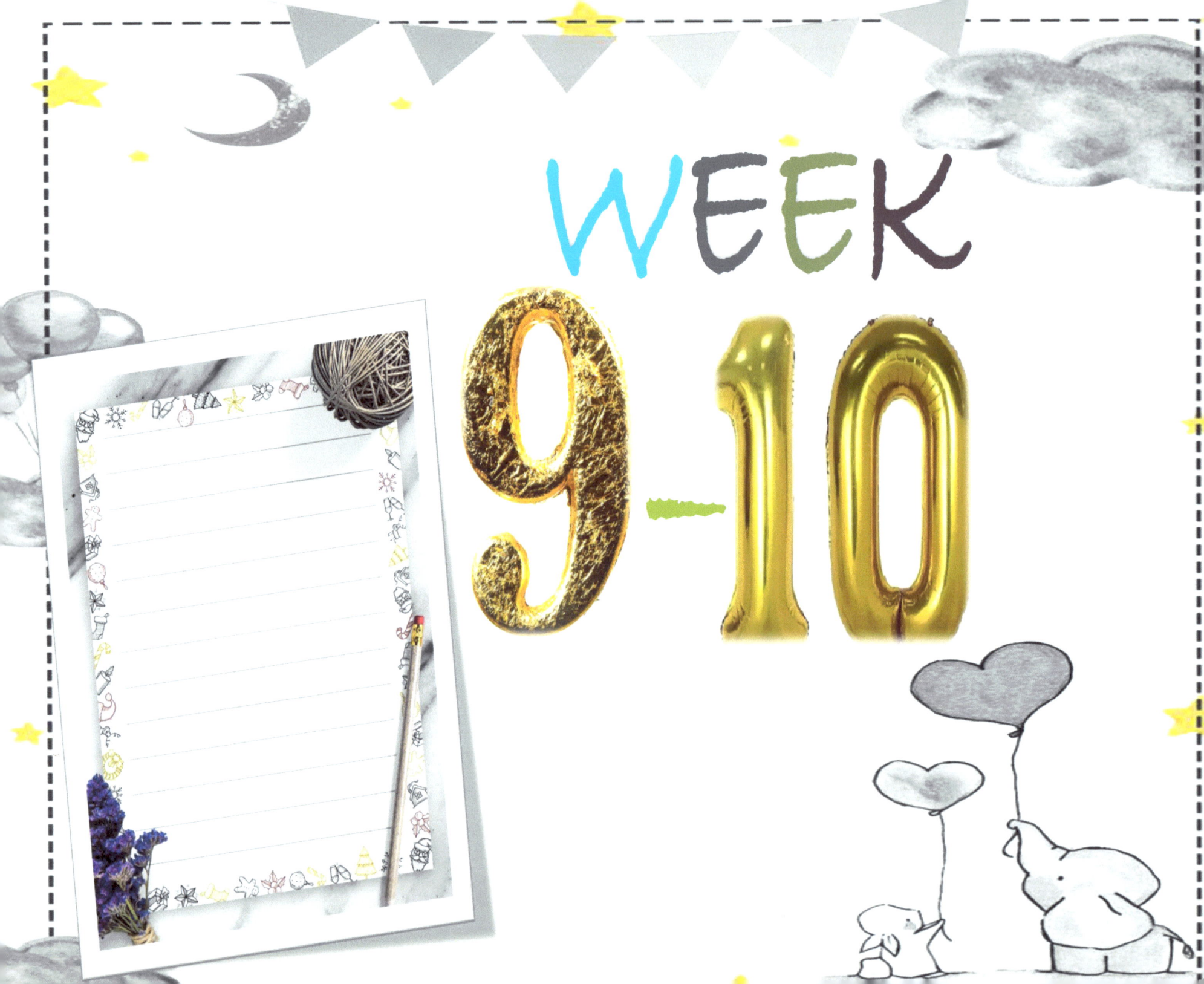

GET YOUR SLEEP

- Sleeping on your left side is ideal for your baby.
- This position allows for maximum blood flow to placenta.
- Sleeping flat can increase your acidity and decrease blood flow to your baby
- Don't lie down immediately after eating. Try walk slowly for 10-15 min after a meal.

HEART BURN & INDIGESTION

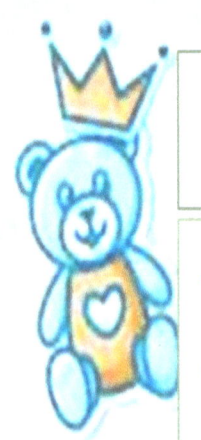
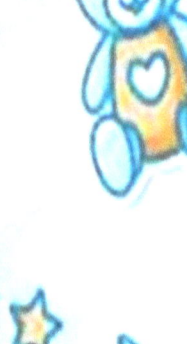
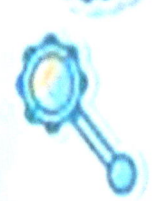
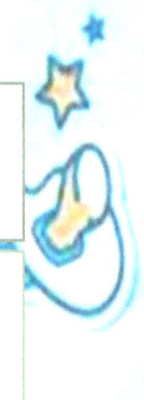
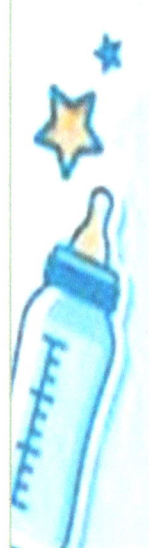

- Have a feeling of acidity? Avoid oil and spicy food.
- Have 6 small meals instead of 3 large ones & try not to sleep or lie down for at least a few hours after your finish meals.
- Increase your water intake.
- Reduce intake of tea, coffee and aerated drinks.
- Increases fruits and vegetables intake.
- Empty stomach produces more acidity.
- Consult your doctor for further medication if the problem persists.

PASTE

YOUR

PICTURE

Write your experiences

HAIR CARE IN PREGNANCY

Second Trimester

Moisturize: Use a pregnancy-safe hair conditioner or natural oils to keep your hair hydrated and reduce frizz. Avoid products containing potentially harmful ingredients like formaldehyde or phthalates.

Heat Styling Precautions: Minimize the use of heat styling tools like straighteners or curling irons, as they can cause damage to your hair. If you do use them, apply a heat protectant spray beforehand.

Regular Trims: Schedule regular hair trims to keep split ends in check and promote healthier hair growth.

SKIN CARE IN PREGNANCY

Second Trimester

Stretch Mark Prevention: As your body undergoes changes, apply a moisturizing lotion or oil to areas prone to stretch marks, such as the belly, breasts, and thighs. Look for products containing ingredients like cocoa butter, shea butter, or vitamin E.

Exfoliation: Gently exfoliate your skin once or twice a week to remove dead skin cells and promote a healthy glow. Opt for mild exfoliants, such as those with fruit enzymes or gentle scrubs, avoiding harsh chemical exfoliants.

Eye Care: Use a hydrating and gentle eye cream to combat puffiness and reduce the appearance of dark circles.

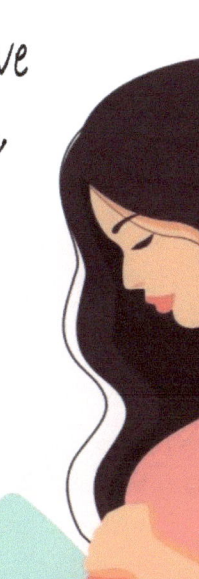

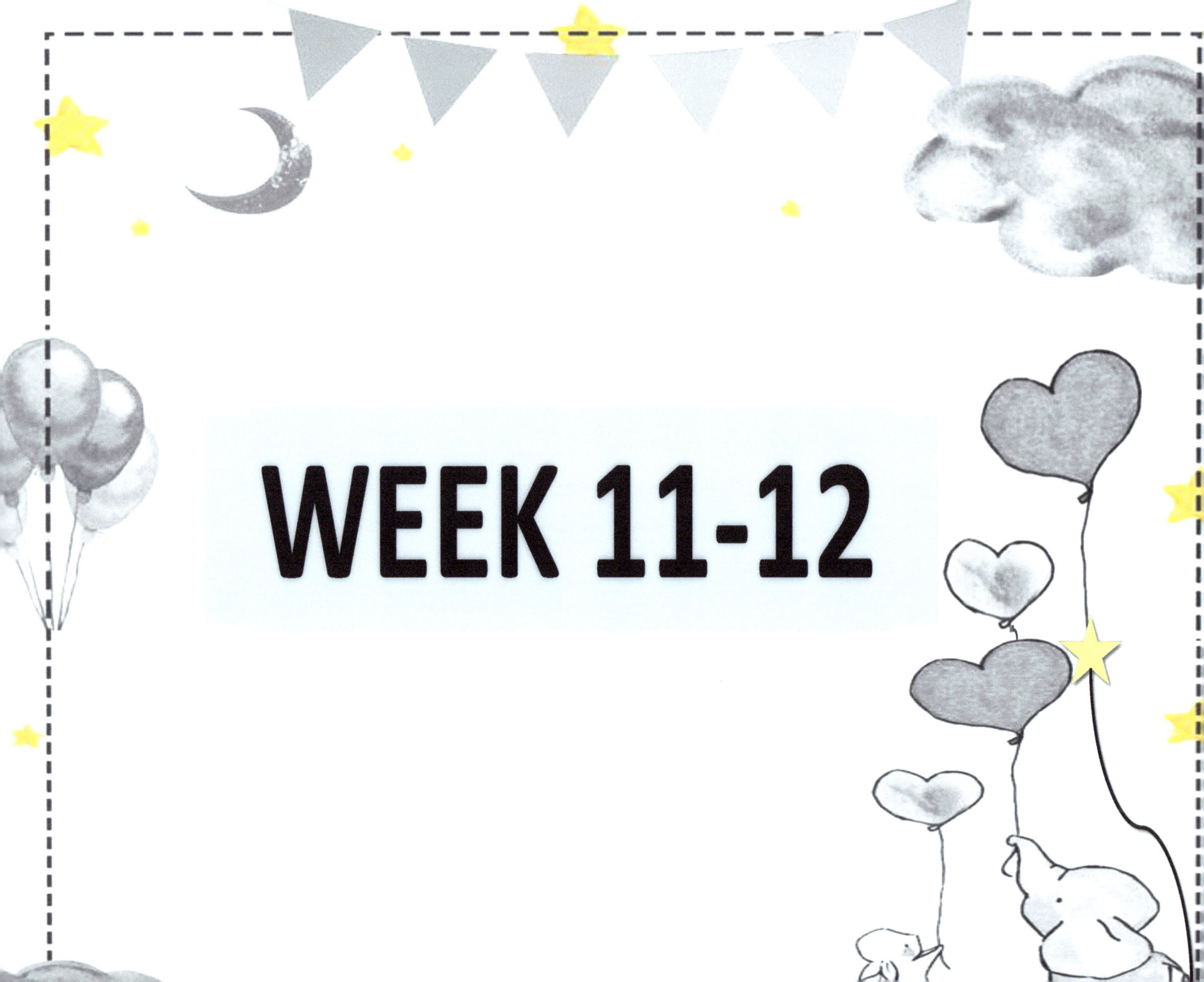

USG PICTURES

USG PICTURES

WEIGHT AND YOGA

- Although a normal weight gain of 10-12 kg is expected during the period of the next 7 months. Its important to know that excess weight gain can be harmful for your health.

- Make sure you keep moving your body. Light exercises like yoga & walking should be performed regularly. Make sure that if you perform weight or intensity exercise. It should be under guidance of certified instructor.

LEG CRAMPS

- If you feel sudden pain in the calves while sleeping, you might be experiencing a cramp. You can reduce the episodes by doing calf stretches.

- Try these foot exercises:

- Bend and stretch your foot up and down 30 times. Rotate your foot 8 times one way and 8 times the other way repeat with other foot. It may help to ease cramp if you pull your toes up towards your ankle or rub the muscle.

- Tip: Keeping yourself hydrated.

EXERCISE IN PREGNANCY

Weeks 13-16

Continue with low-impact exercises and gradually increase your activity level as tolerated. Consider incorporating exercises specifically targeting the pelvic floor muscles, such as Kegels, to strengthen the pelvic area and prepare for childbirth.

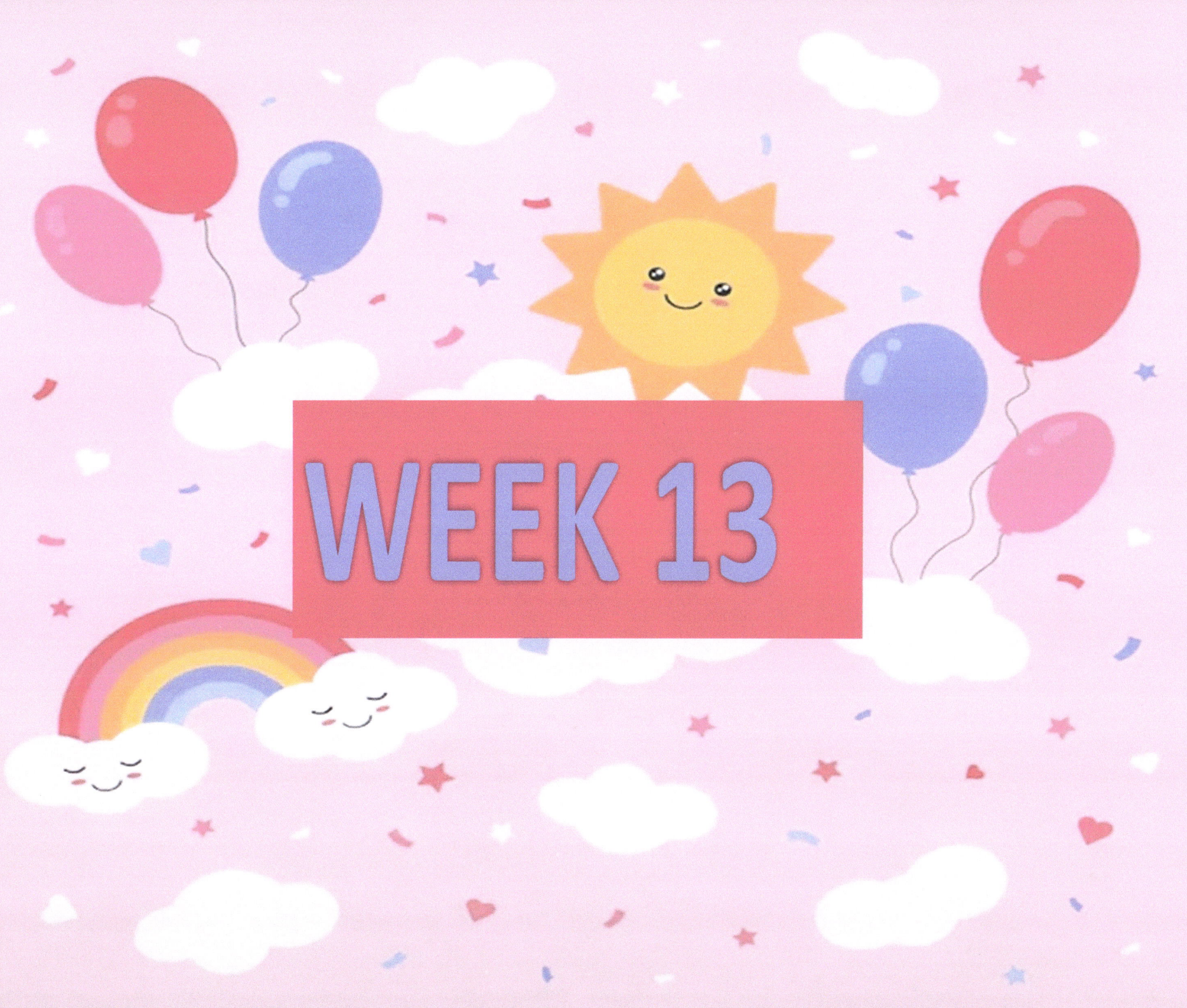

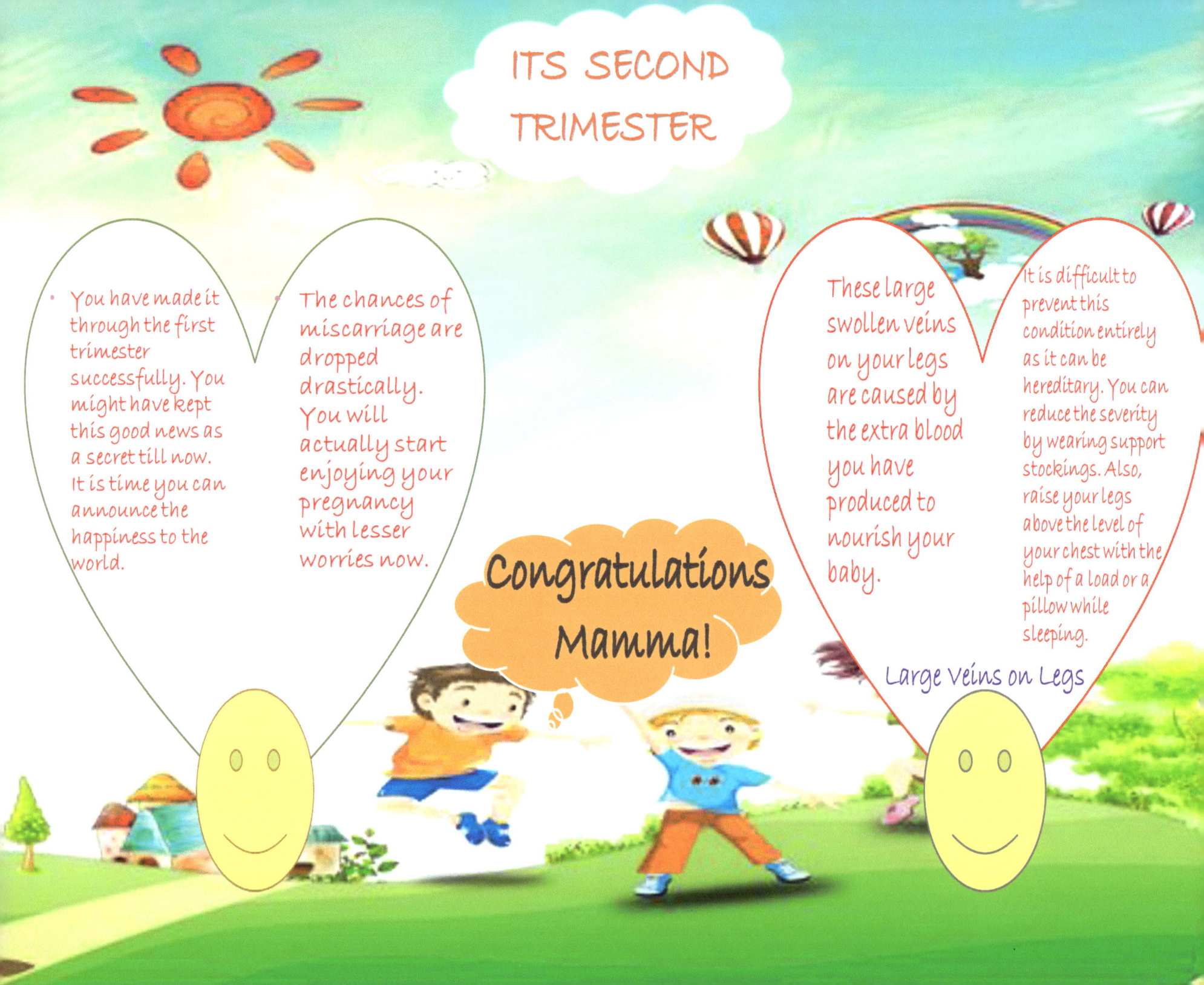

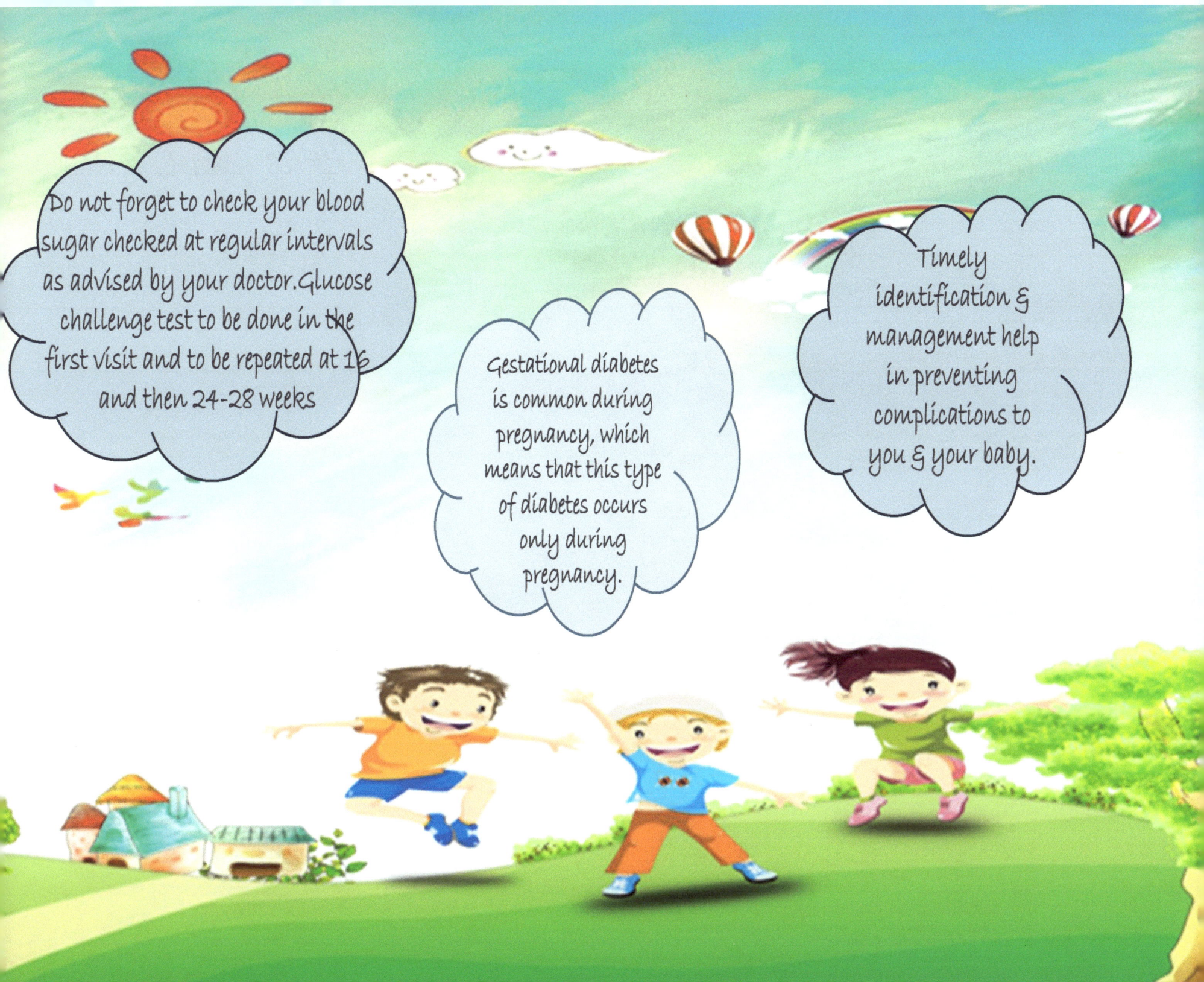

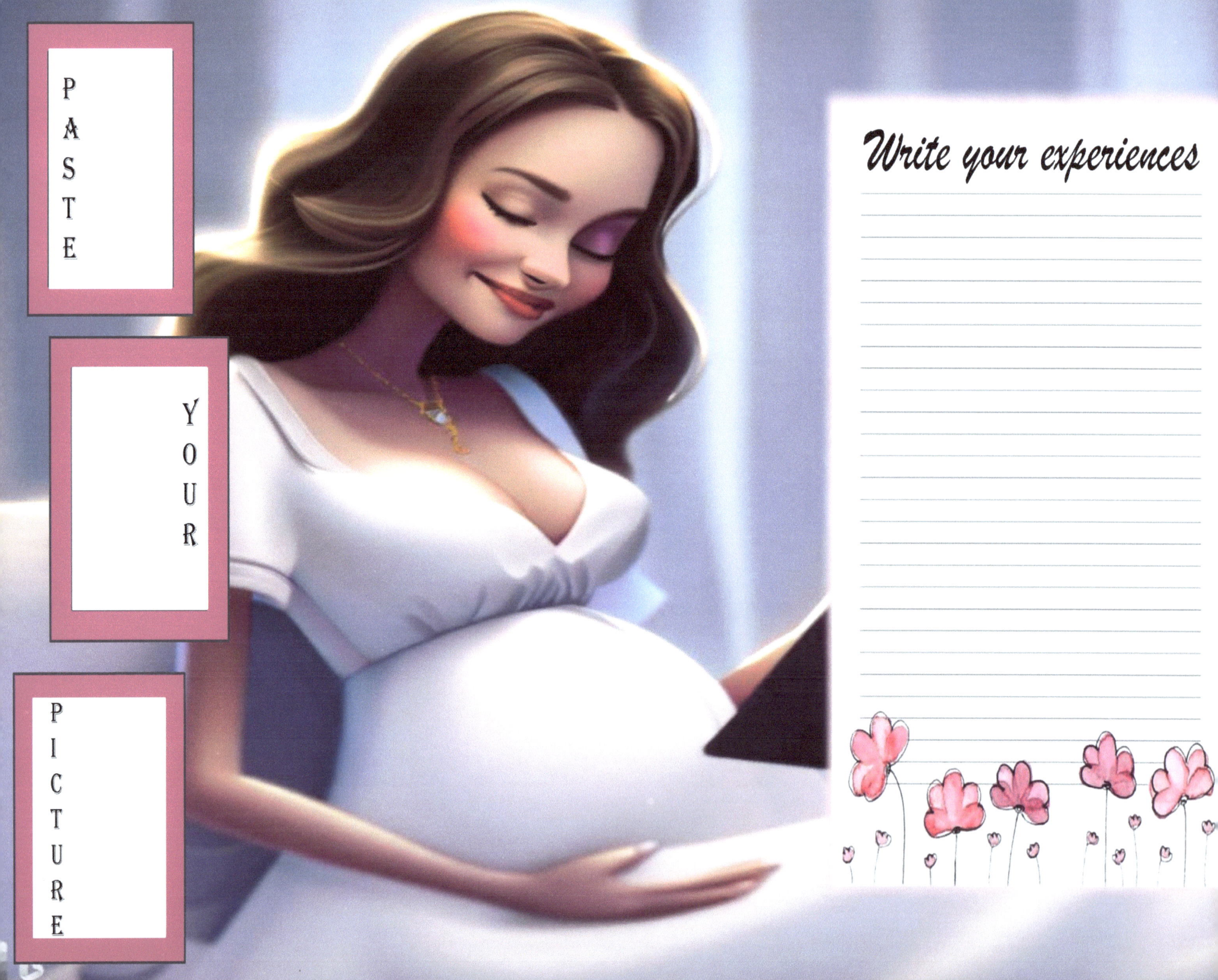

WEEK 14

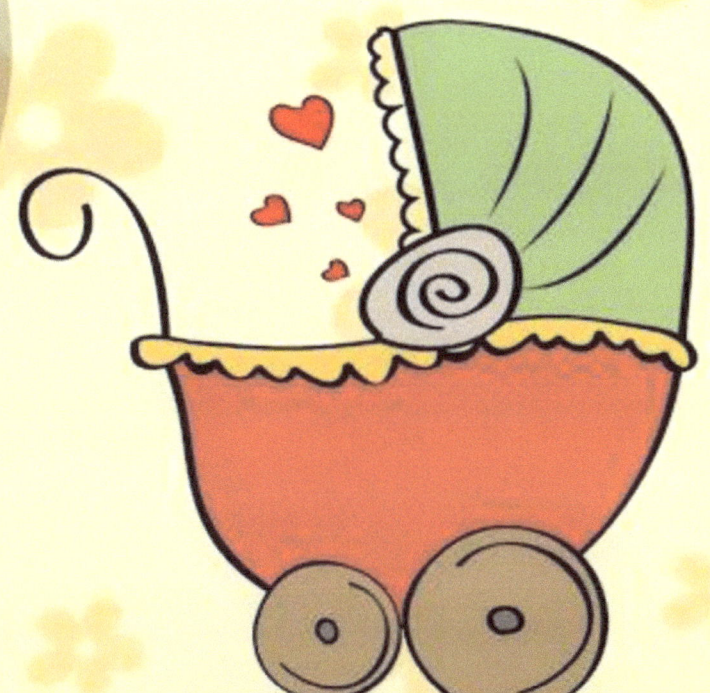

BLEEDING GUMS

Have you noticed that your gums are bleeding after brushing? This due to those pregnancy hormones! While this is normal, it's an important to keep brushing regularly.

Also, sees the dentist at least once during pregnancy to avoid gum disease, which can cause pregnancy complications like preterm labour if untreated

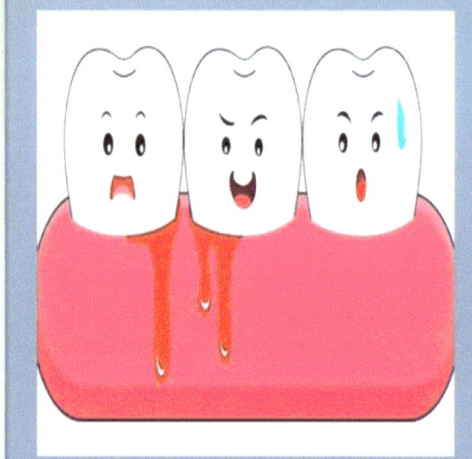

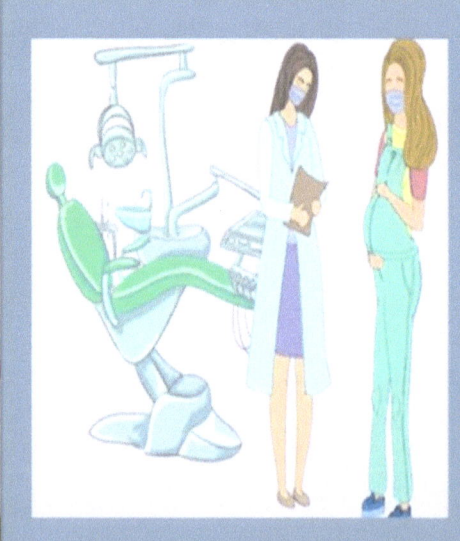

PREGNANCY DONT'S

- Do not fast or stay hungry for more than 4-6 hours as it can cause decrease in glucose levels in the blood this reduces the energy supply to the baby & is not recommended.
- Tip: Cut down the intake of tea, coffee and chocolates which triggers burning sensation in your chest. Taking tea just after meal decreases the absorption of iron too

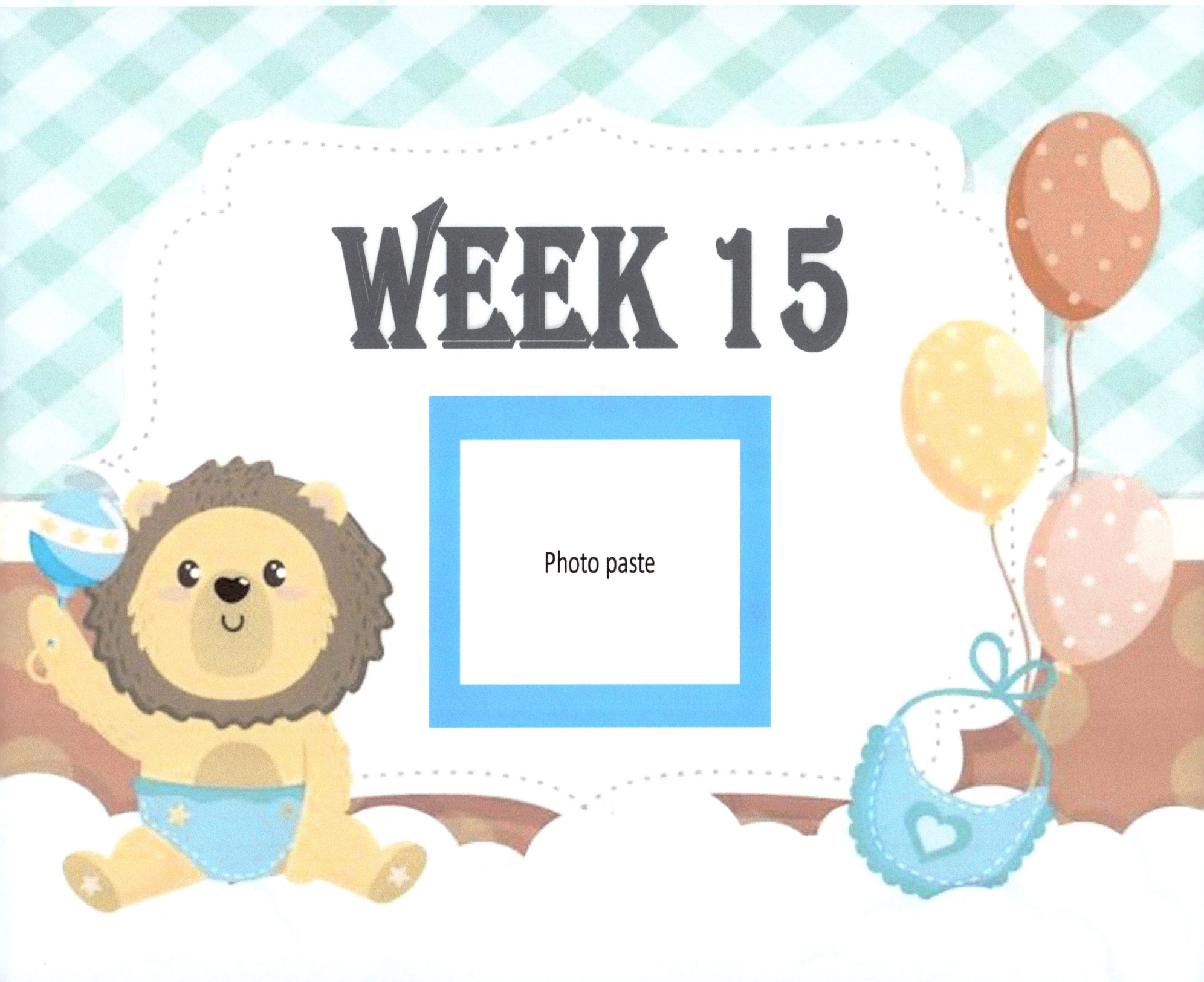

TRAVELLING DURING PREGNANCY

- The most viable and safe time to travel during pregnancy is between 14th-28th weeks.

- While travelling by road/air or other ways of transport a seat belt should always be worn the belts should be snug but not uncomfortable or tight.

- The Safest mode of travel is by train.

- Air travel should not be done in third trimester and if there are complications like placenta previa, pregnancy induced hypertension and sickle cell disease

PASTE

YOUR

PICTURE

Write your experiences

WEEK 16

BACKACHES

TRY THESE TIPS

- Bend your knees and keep your back straight when you lift or pick something up from the floor.
- Avoid lifting heavy objects
- Move your feet when you turn to avoid twisting spine.
- Wear flat shoes to evenly distribute your weight.
- Keep your back straight and well supported when sitting - look for maternity support pillows.
- Use a mattress that supports you properly - you can put a piece of hardboard under a soft mattress to make it firmer, if necessary.
- Try to balance the weight between 2 bags when carrying shopping.
- Get enough rest, particularly later in pregnancy

PREGNANCY ESSENTIALS

The following are some essential items for the second trimester of your pregnancy

- PILLOWS
- PEPPERMINT OIL FOR NAUSEA
- HEATING PAD
- LOOSE CLOTHES
- STAY HYDRATED
- KEEP ALL MEDICINES HANDY
- MOISTURIZER

EXERCISE IN PREGNANCY

Weeks 17-20

Continue with low-impact cardio exercises like walking or swimming. Incorporate exercises that improve posture and strengthen the back, such as prenatal Pilates or yoga. Focus on gentle stretches and exercises that alleviate common discomforts like lower back pain and joint stiffness.

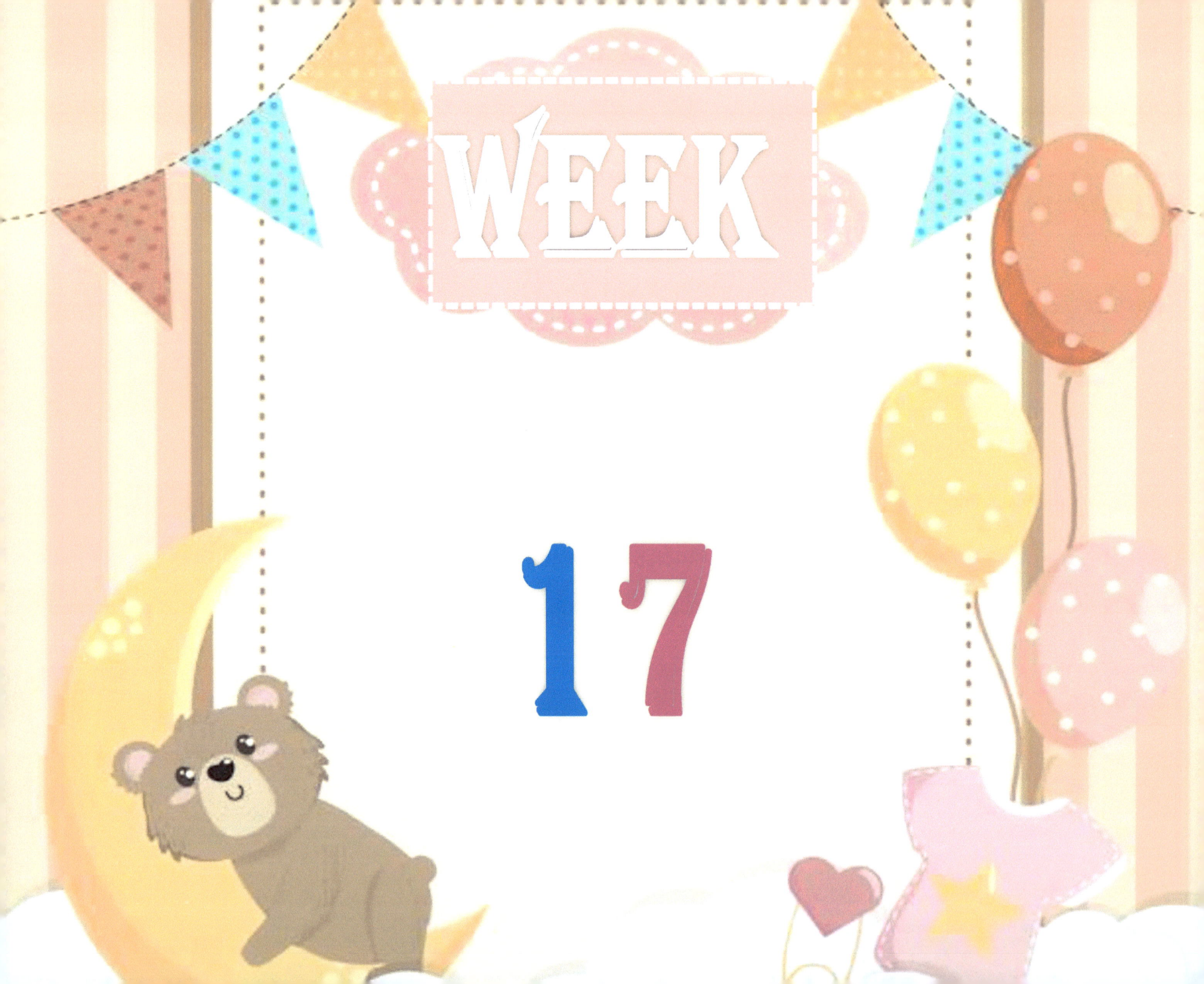

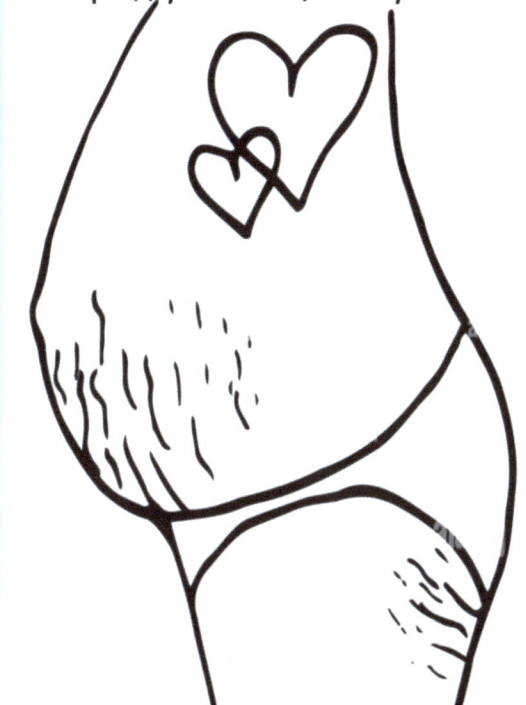

STRETCH MARKS

https://youtu.be/llOhlyNXNZE

Don't worry as it is common. The good news is that stretch marks usually became considerably less noticeable about 6 to 12 months after childbirth. Keep the skin well-nourished, coconut oil is the best.

If you gain weight slowly with proper diet and exercise, the stretching becomes gradual. Don't worry about stretch mark LASER is becoming very promising in stretch mark removal. Ask your doctor about it.

They are common in pregnancy, affecting around 8 out of 10 pregnant women. They usually appear on your tummy, or sometimes on your upper thighs and breasts, as your pregnancy progresses and your bump starts to grow.

Pregnancy Weight Gain

	Pre-pregnancy BMI [kg/m²]	Recommended pregnancy weight gain [kg]
Underweight	<18.5	12.5–18
Normal weight	19–24.9	11.5–16
Overweight	25–29.9	7–11.5
Obese	>30	5–9

ACOG 2009

What's Normal?

- In first three months : 1 to 1.5 kg.
- In second and third trimester: 5kg each
- Ideal Weight Gain: 11.5 to 16kg

CAN BABIES HEAR INSIDE THE WOMB?

- Cells that form ears develop at 4-5th week.

- Your baby forms tools to hear in the 18th week.

- Can hear your heartbeat and breath

- Baby can start hearing in third trimester.

- Your voice is the first thing your baby hears; outside noises are muffled.

Read the books you love, listen to the music which soothe your soul. Moral values can be imprinted in the babys mind at this very time as per ongoing researches.

RELAX AND TAKE REST

- Always remember to relax and take rest. It is very important for you and your baby.

- Sleep on the left side to reduce pressure on back veins and improve blood supply to your heart.

PASTE YOUR PICTURE

Write your experiences

WEEK 18

Photo paste

HAVE A WALK!

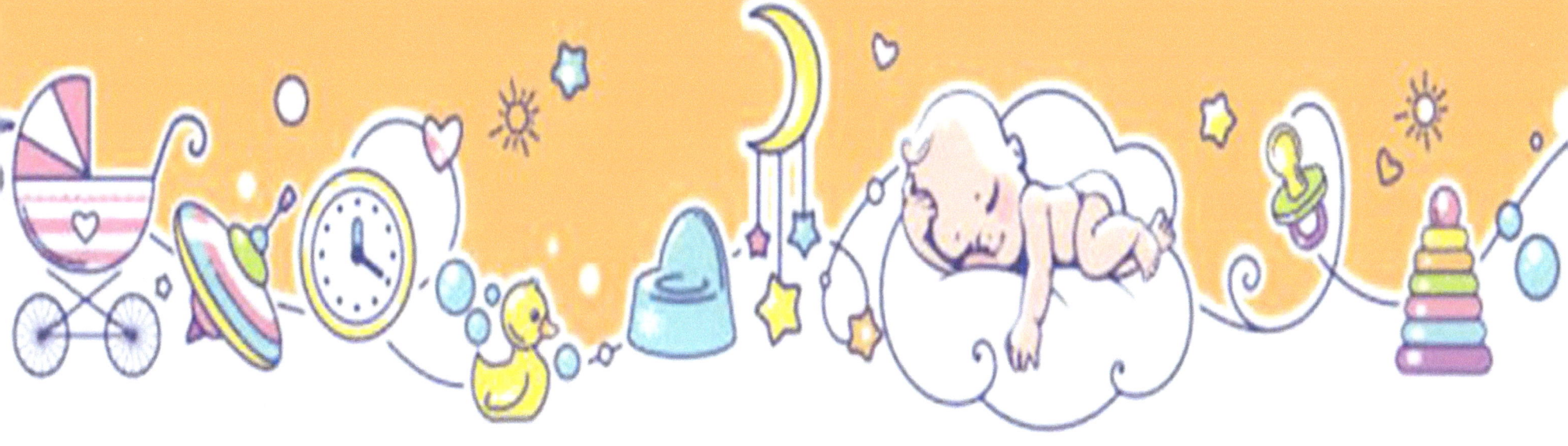

- Make sure you get a limited amount of physical activity daily.
- The best way is following a fixed time for walk- rather than waiting for some free time.
- Choose a ventilated space (mostly around nature) for a walk.
- Remember to keep yourself hydrated after the exercise.

Having Swelling in Feet?

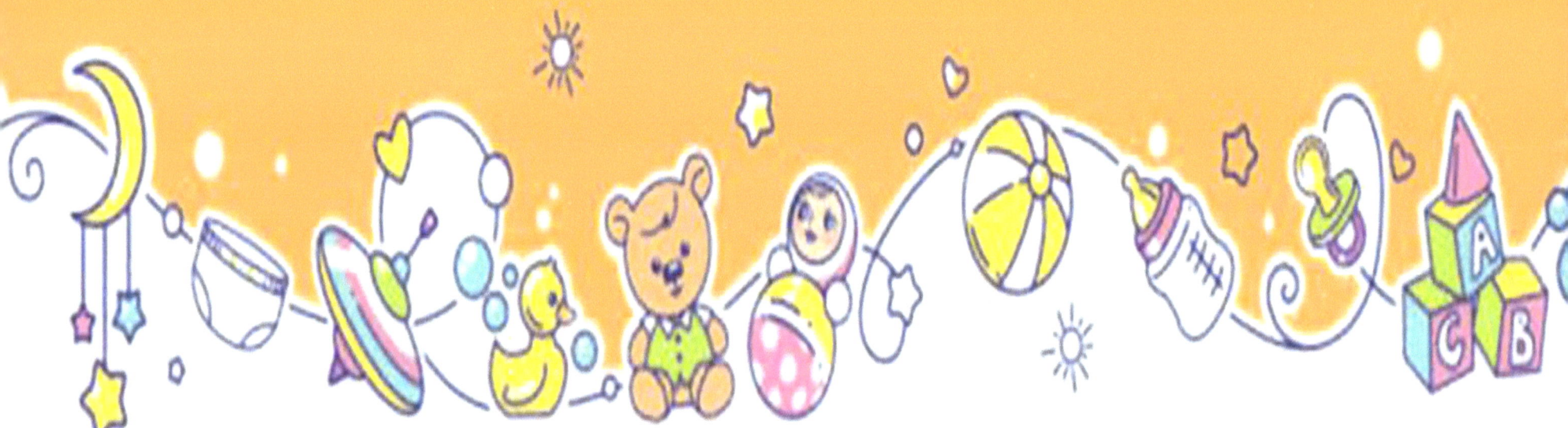

Swelling of feet in ankle usually confined to one leg, more on right, disappears on rest alone and if not associated with other pregnancy complications is called physiological edema. Discuss about it with your doctor and don't worry. This is due to increase venous pressure caused by growing uterus. Abdomen or genital area needs urgent attention. A good warning sign can be abnormal tightening of ring on the figure.

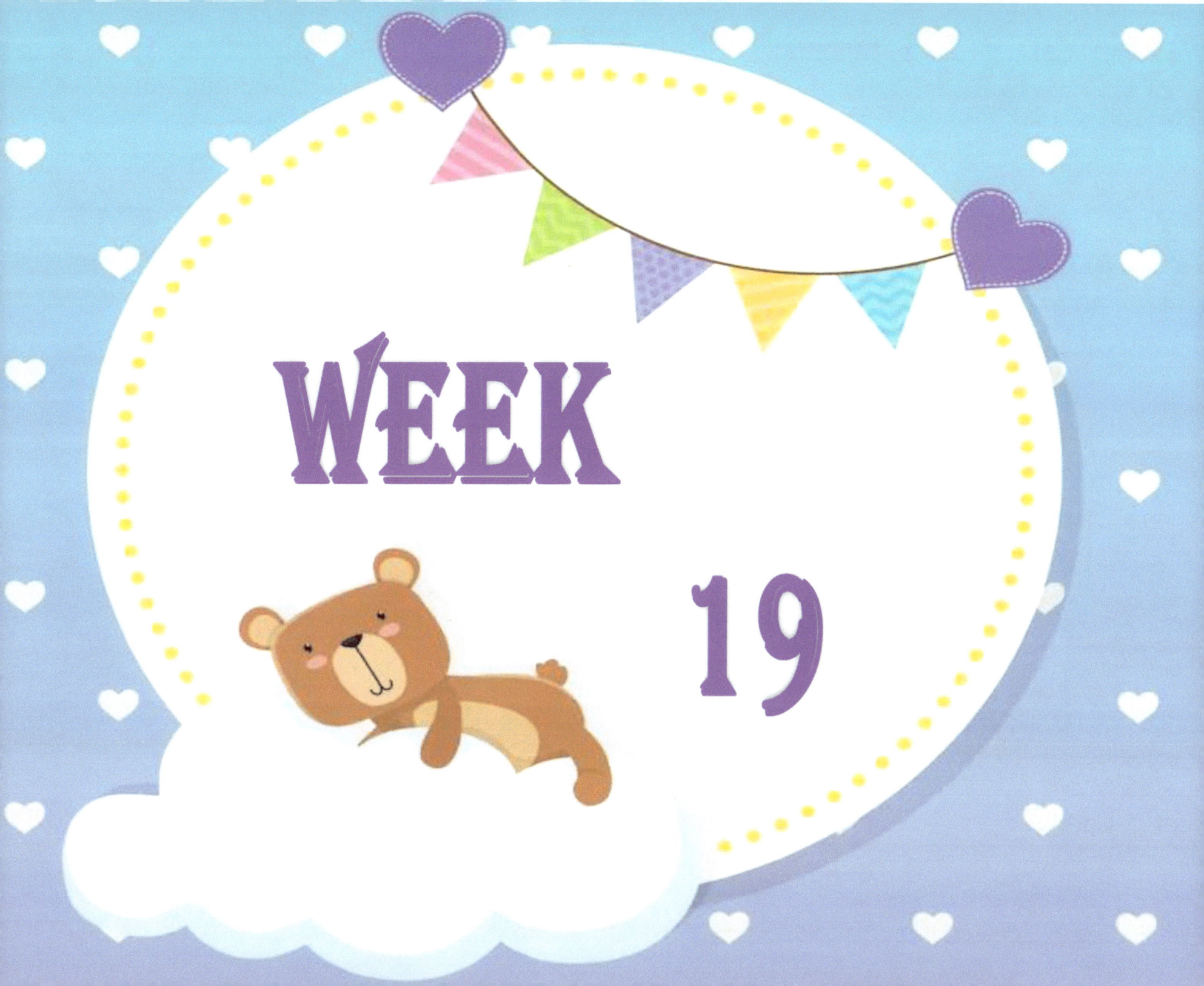

EMBRACE SELF CARE

Tips

- Utilize this good phase for indulging in your hobby for some creativity.
- Give oil massage to the body followed by a hot water bath.
- Read good books to improve your concentration.
- Talk your body, it will make you feel happier and less stressed.

Feeling Hot Flushes in pregnancy?

- You're likely to feel warmer than usual during pregnancy. This is due to hormonal changes and an increase in blood supply to the skin. You're also likely to sweat more.

- It can help you.

- Wear loose clothing made of natural fibers, as these are more absorbent and breathable than synthetic fibers.

- Keep your room cool- you could use an electric fan.

- Wash face frequently to help you feel fresh.

- Don't exert too much.

- You can use steam to get relief from blocked nose. Practicing breathing.

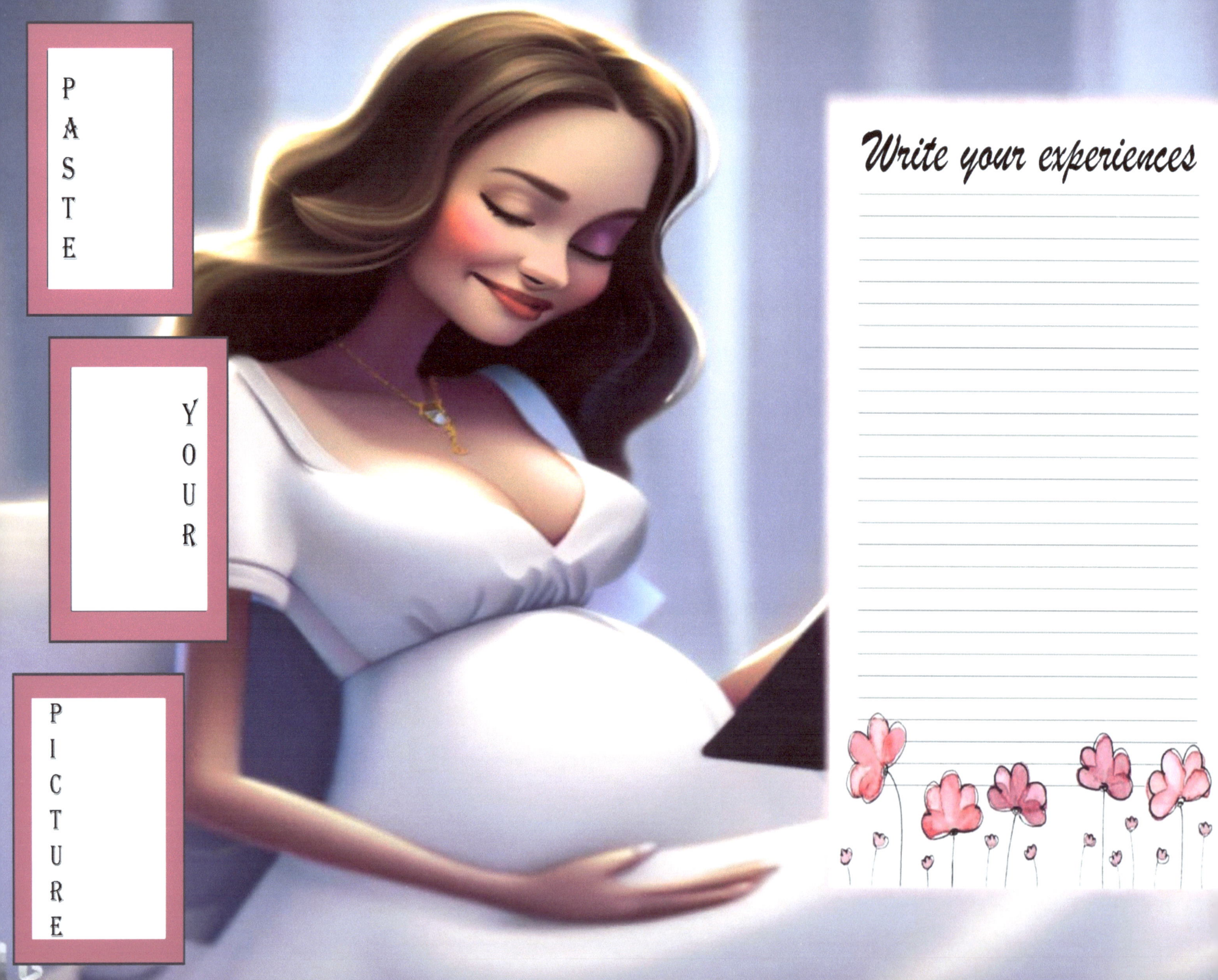

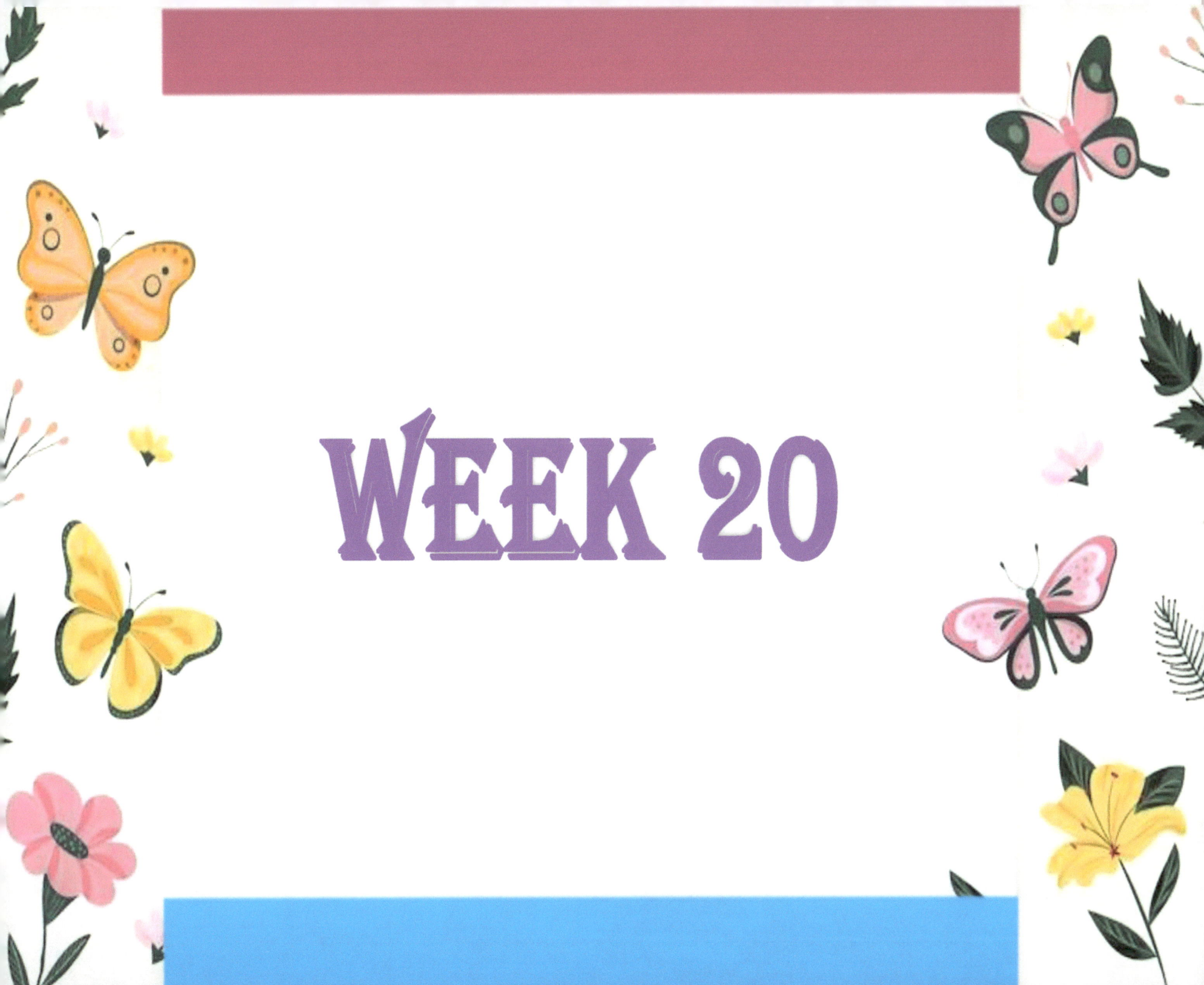

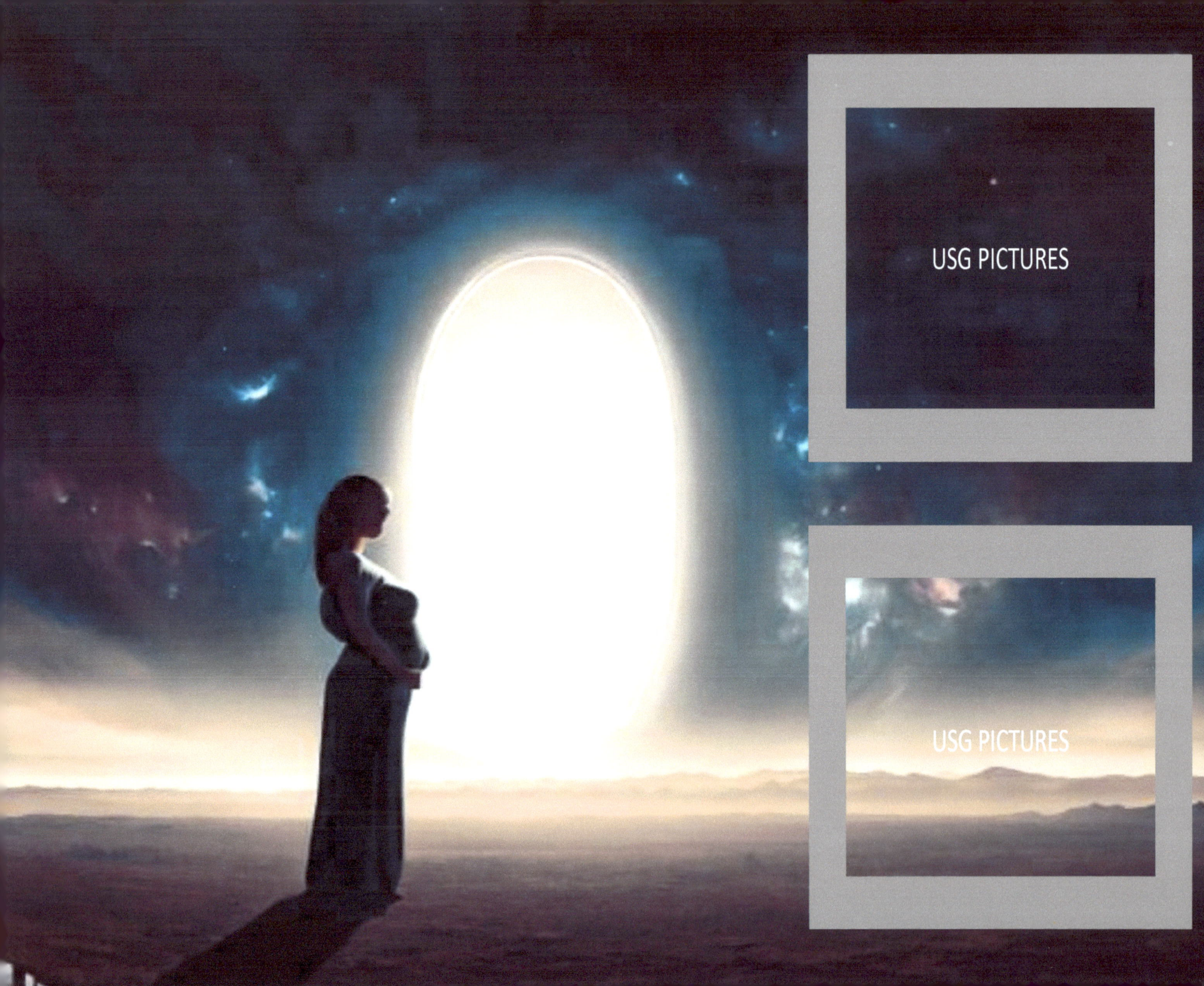

BREAST CARE

- It is important to begin preparing the breast for breastfeeding during the prenatal period. Post the fourth month some secretions might be there leaving the breasts itchy and damp.

- Washing is the basic form of hygiene and is to done without soap to remove secretions, and lanolin must be applied after to prevent evaporation of perspiration and softening the skin.

- A well fitted support bra should be worn at all times to support the enlarging the breast.

TO GET GOOD SLEEP

- Avoid tea, coffee or cola drinks in the evening, as caffeine can make it harder to fall a sleep.

- Try bed time medication (Yog Nidra Particularly)

- Try to relax before bedtime so you are not wide awake.

- Exercise can help you have a good sleep, so try to do some activity, such as walk at lunch time or going swimming, even if you feel tired during the stay.

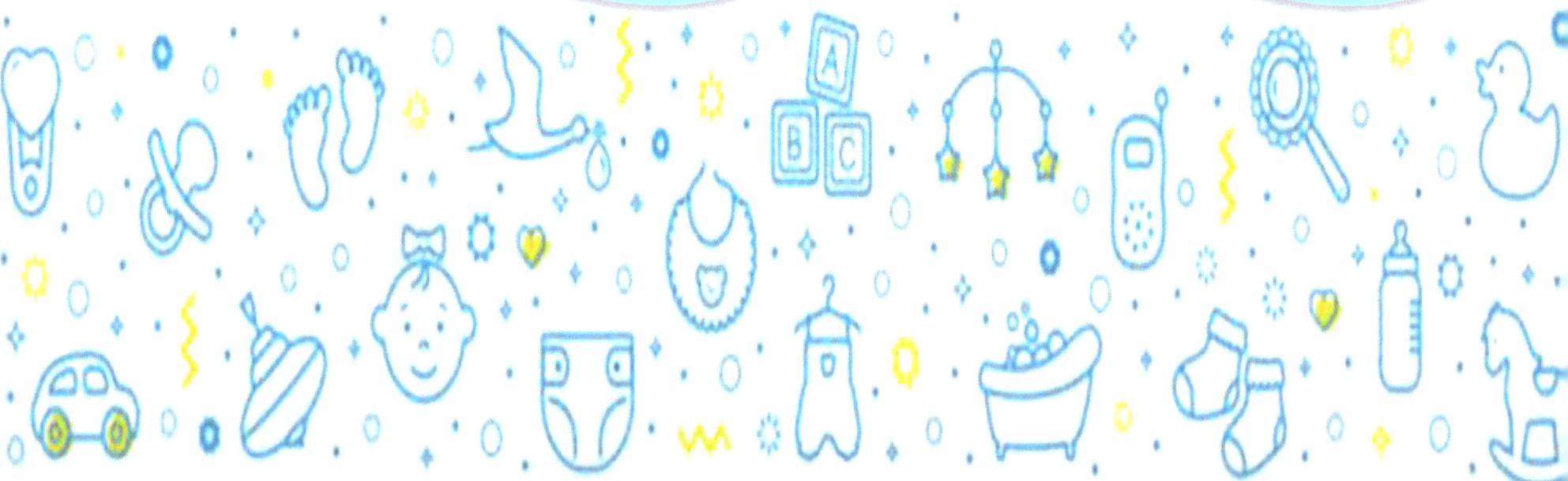

If you don't fall asleep within 15 minutes of retiring to bed then toss & turn on bed, rather get up- sit on sofa, chair etc. and start reading something and when feel drowsy then go to your bed again. Tossing & turning on bed can negatively affect your circadian rhythm of your sleep cycle.

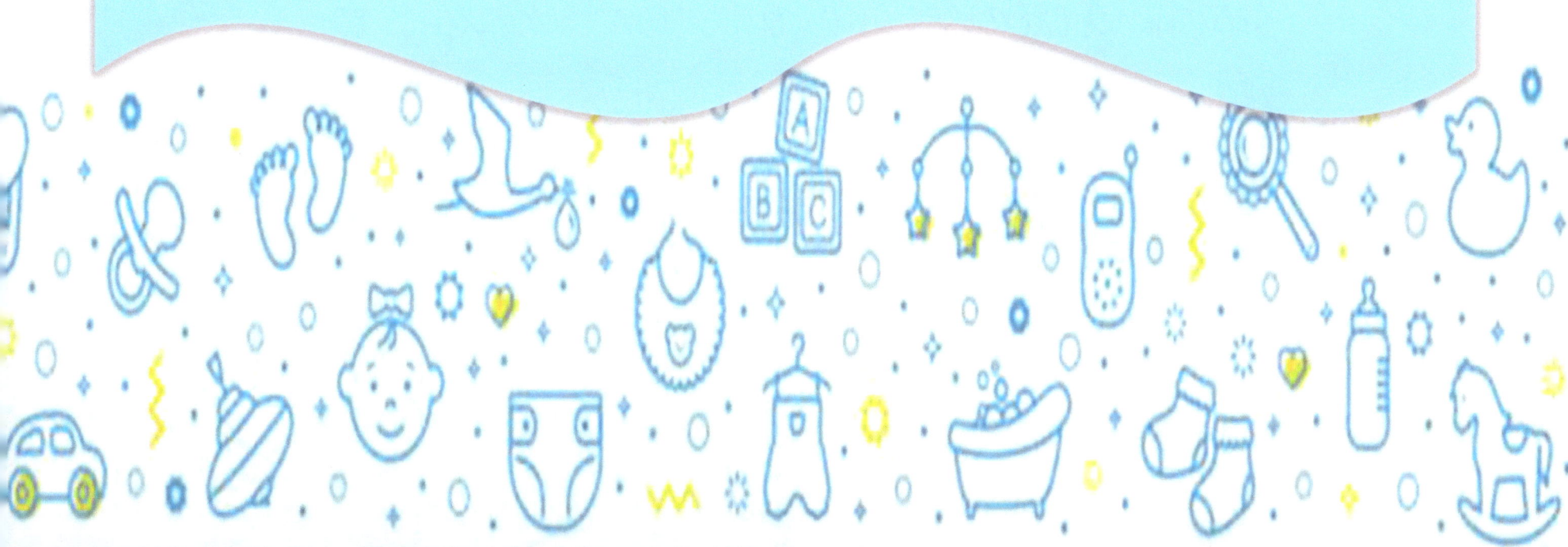

EXERCISE IN PREGNANCY

Weeks 21-24

Maintain your exercise routine and consider adding exercises that help improve balance, such as prenatal yoga or tai chi. Practice deep breathing exercises and relaxation techniques to reduce stress and promote relaxation.

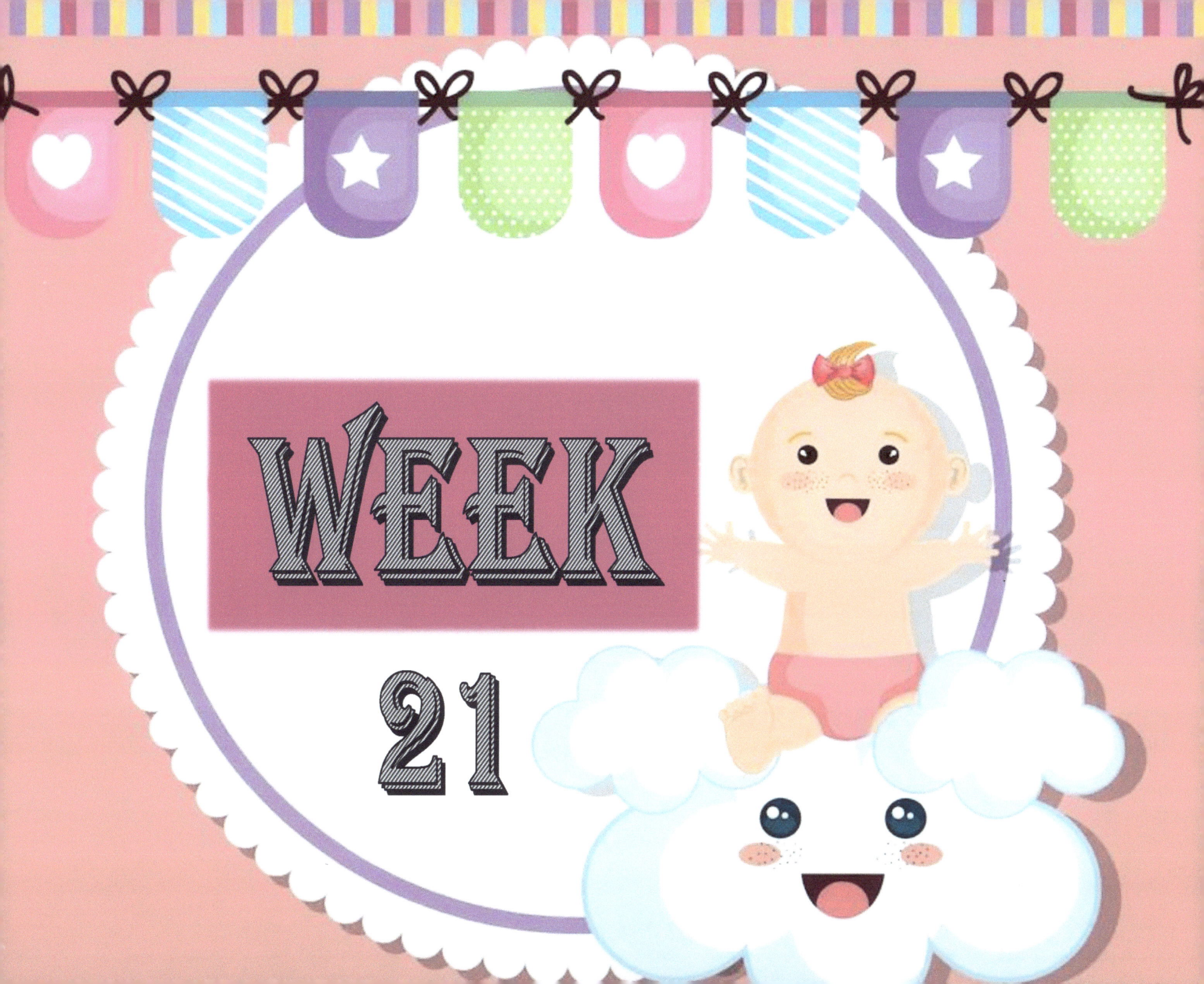

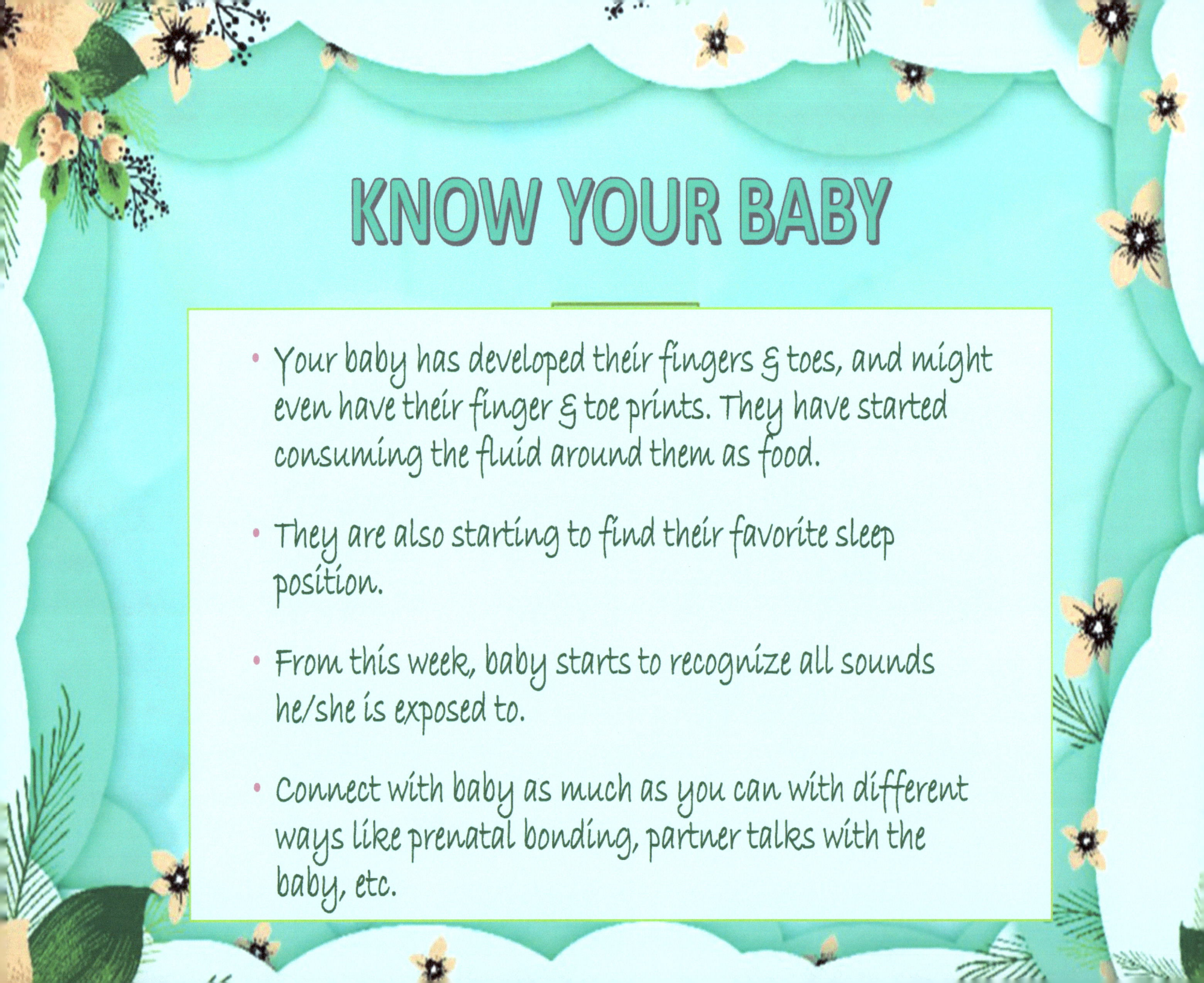

CURB YOUR CRAVINGS

Now your baby is around 600gm, and this rapid growth will increase your hunger, try having healthy options n like vegetables omlet, paranthas & fruits like dates (khajooor), bananas, fig (anjeer), oranges. Increasing your protein intake will help settle your cravings.

- Chana & peanuts
- Makhana (Fox Nuts)
- Almond & raisins
- Roasted paneer
- Coconut water

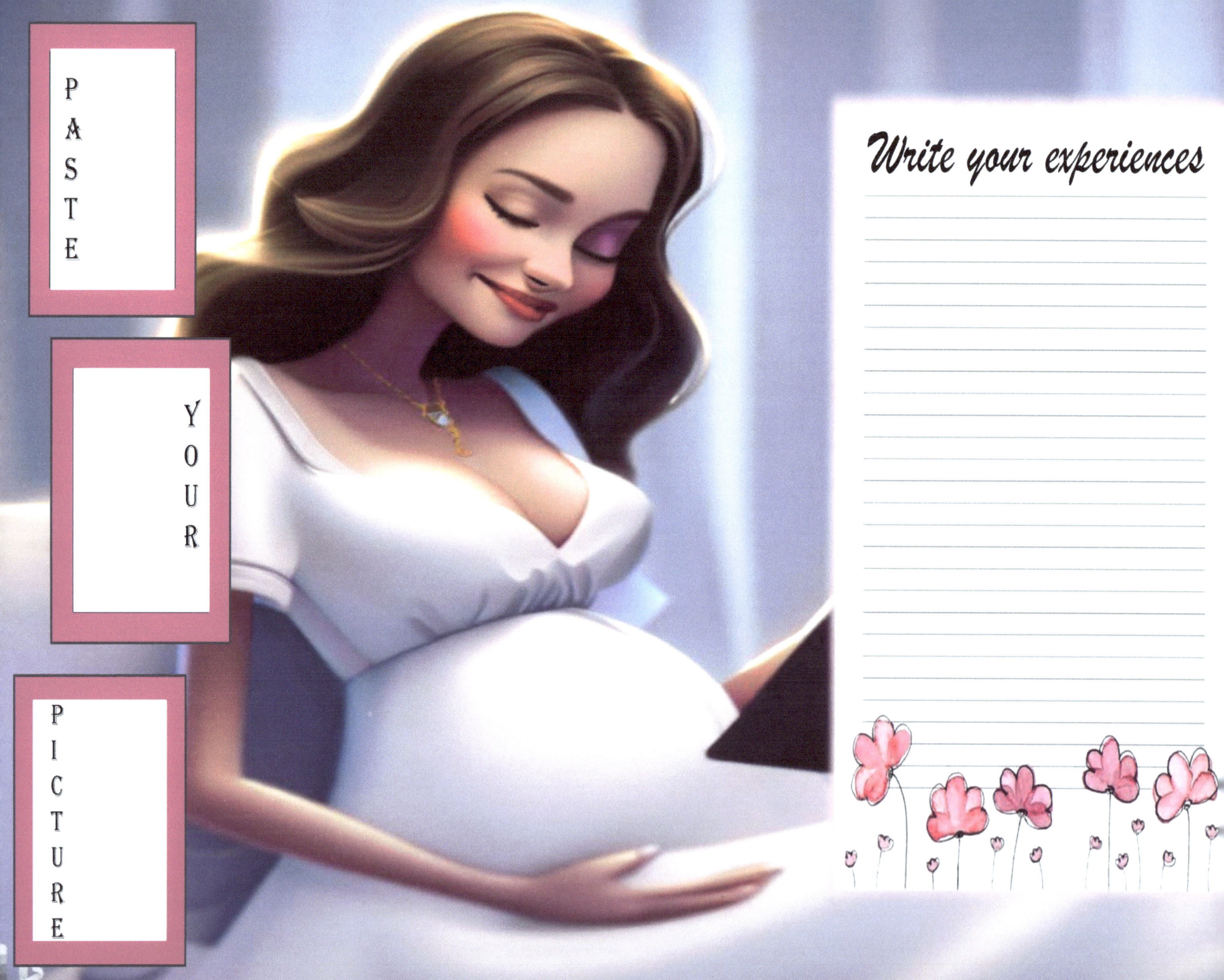

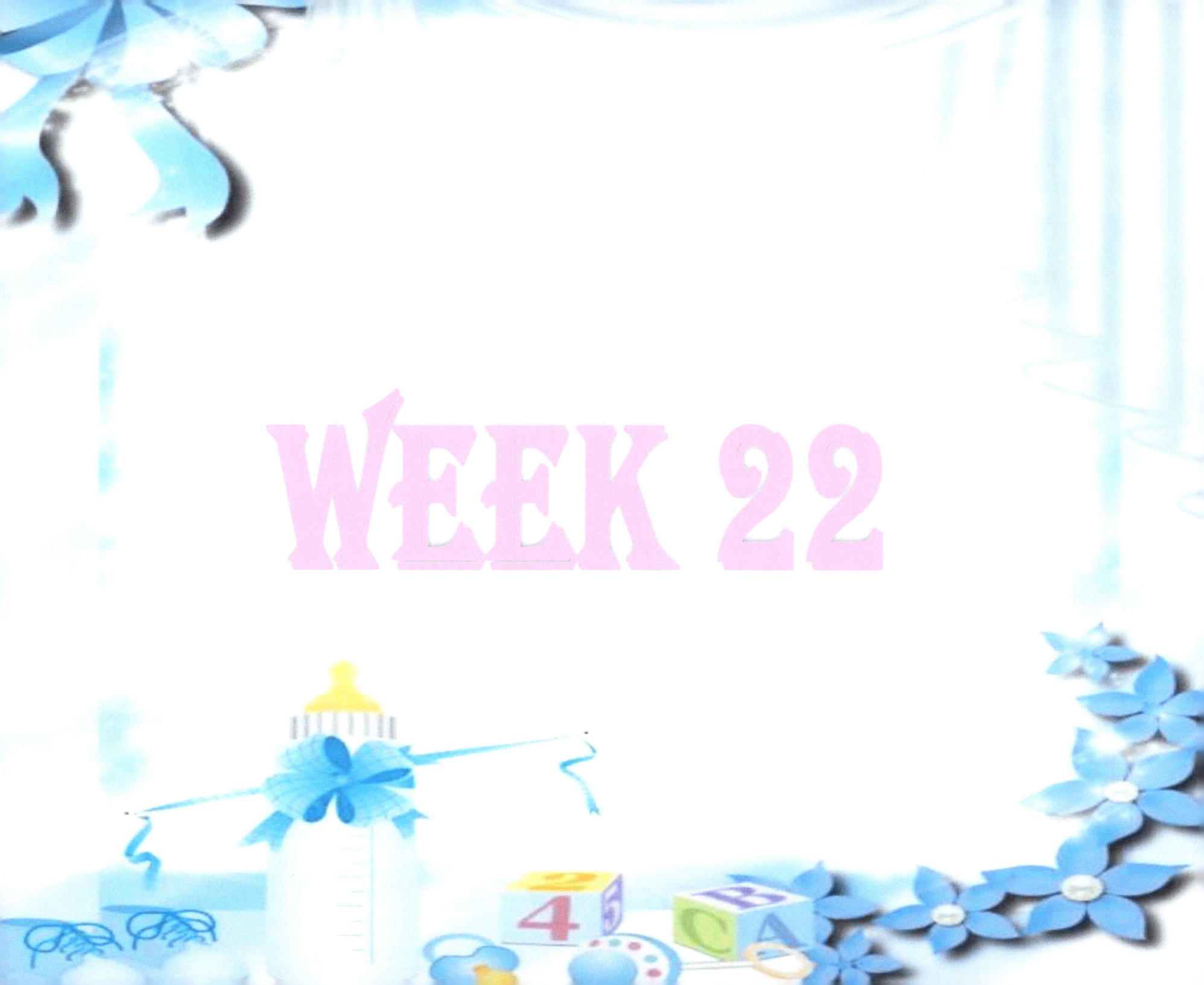

Is your belly button pointing out?

- Don't worry; it is normal during pregnancy for the belly button to point outwards.

- After delivery, it will revert to normal but be prepared for the fact that you will probably left with a slightly larger navel.

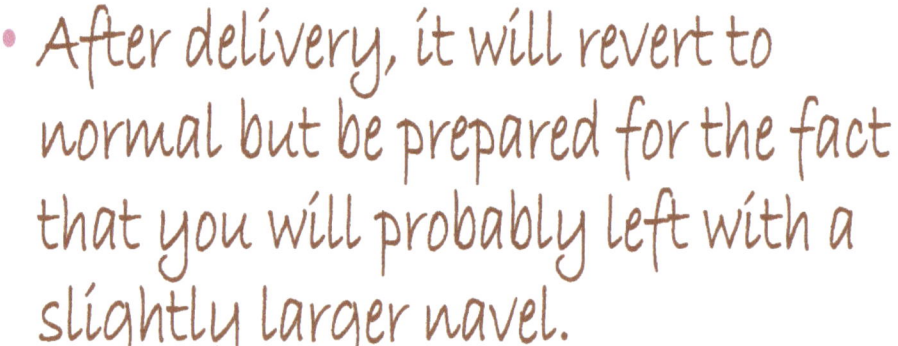
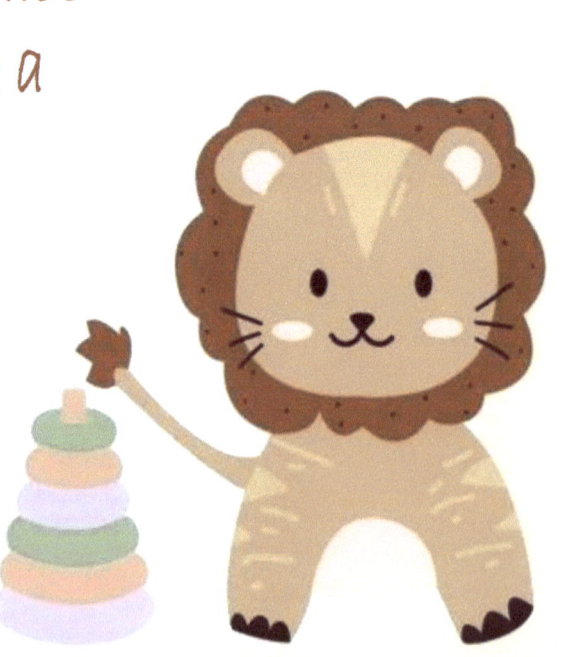

STAYING FIT?

- Join prenatal yoga sessions that are conducted to help you stay fit and active in your pregnancy. It is a gentle and safe way to stretch and strengthen your muscles to support your changing body.

- Benefits of prenatal yoga:

- Improve Sleep

- Reduce stress and anxiety.

- Increase the strength and endurance of muscles needed for normal vaginal delivery.

- Decrease lower back pain, nausea, headache and shortness of breath.

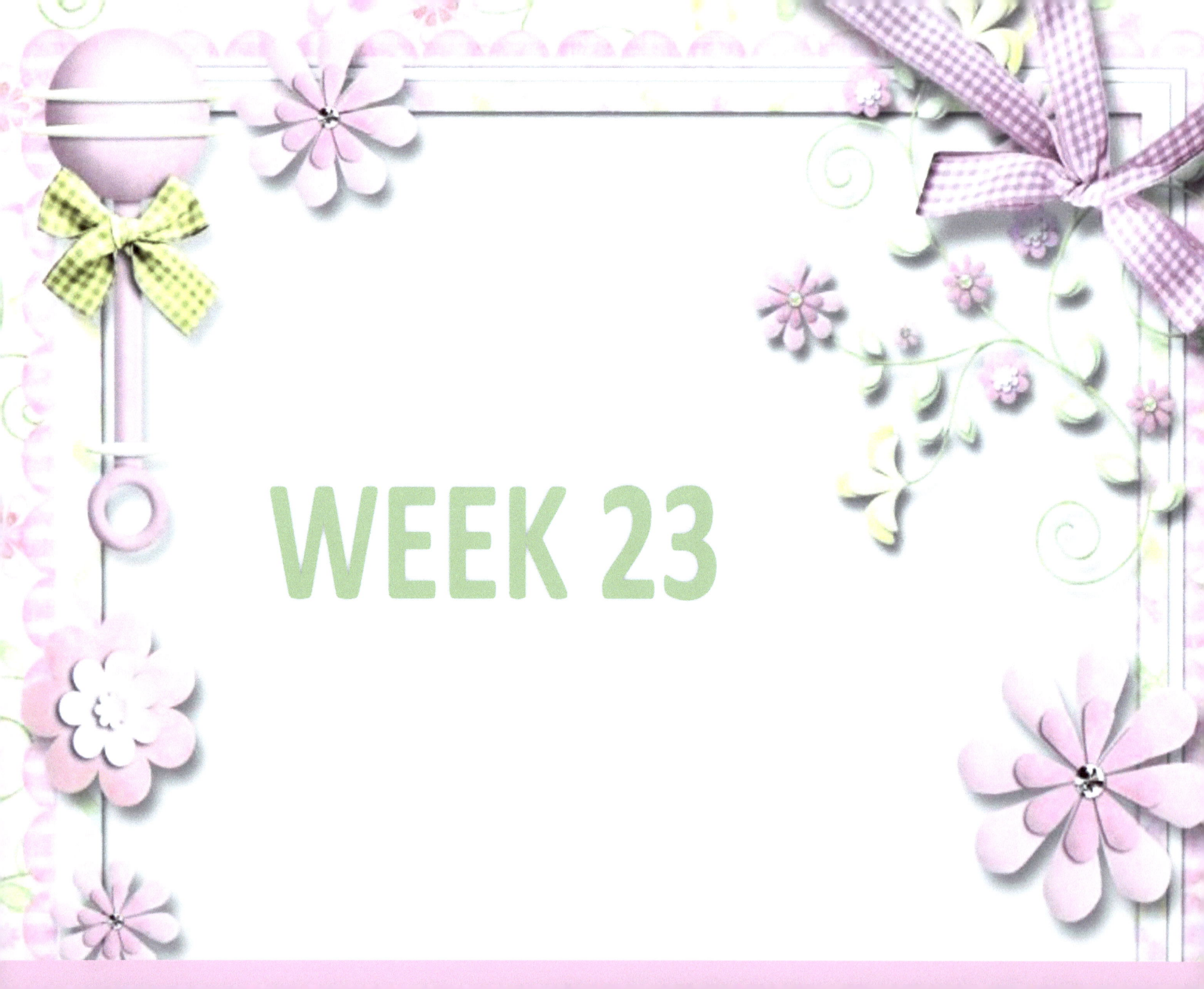

MANAGE BACKACHES

TRY THESE TIPS

- Bend your knees and keep your back straight when you lift or pick something up from the floor.

- Avoid lifting heavy objects.

- Move your feet when you turn to avoid twisting spine.

- Wear flat shoes to evenly distribute your weight.

- Try to balance the weight between 2 bags when carrying shopping.

- Keep your back straight and well supported when sitting-look for maternity support pillows.

- Get enough rest, particularly later in pregnancy.

- Have a massage or a warm bath.

- Use a mattress that supports you properly- you can put a piece of hardboard under a soft mattress to make it firmer, if necessary.

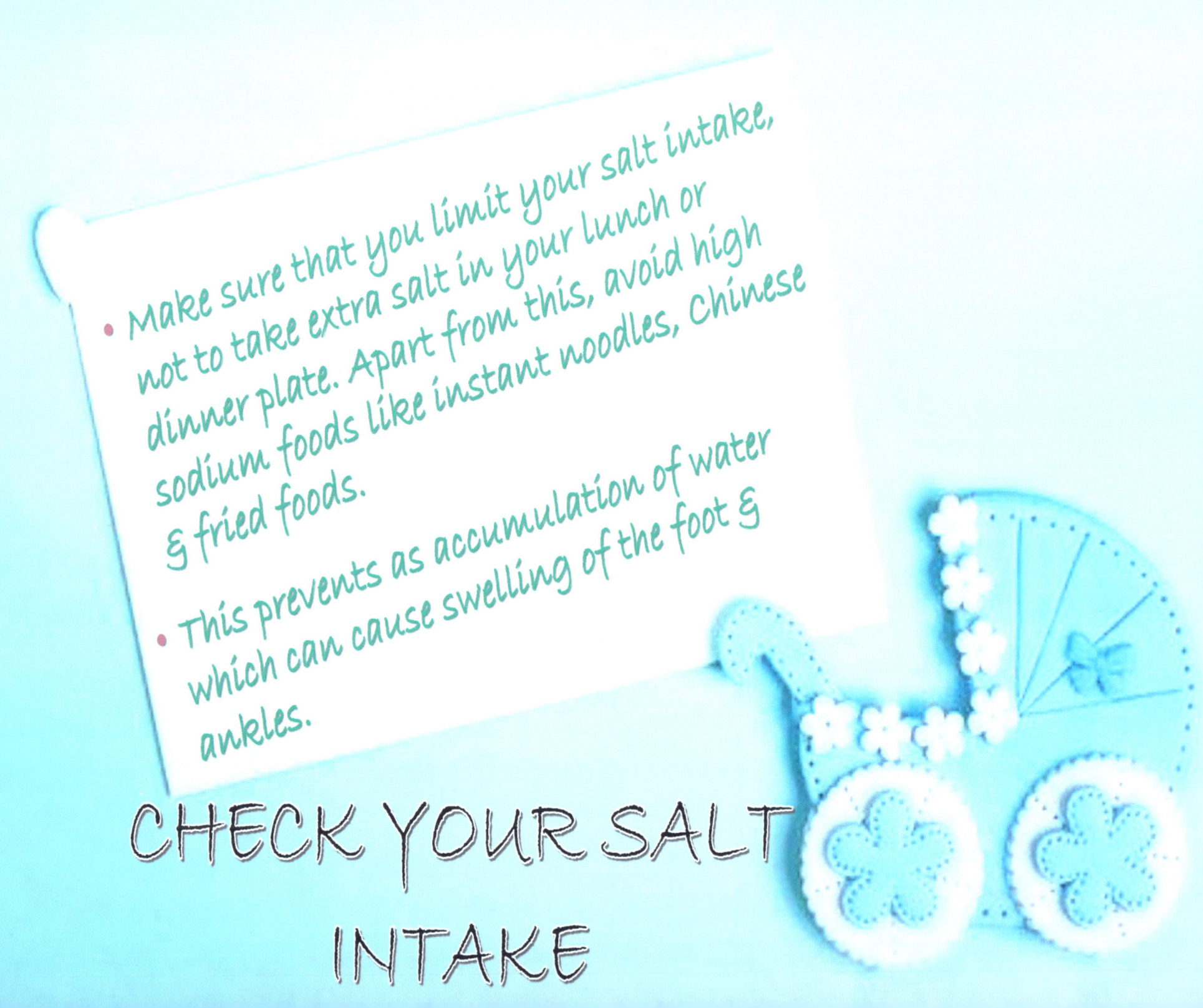

- Make sure that you limit your salt intake, not to take extra salt in your lunch or dinner plate. Apart from this, avoid high sodium foods like instant noodles, Chinese & fried foods.

- This prevents as accumulation of water which can cause swelling of the foot & ankles.

CHECK YOUR SALT INTAKE

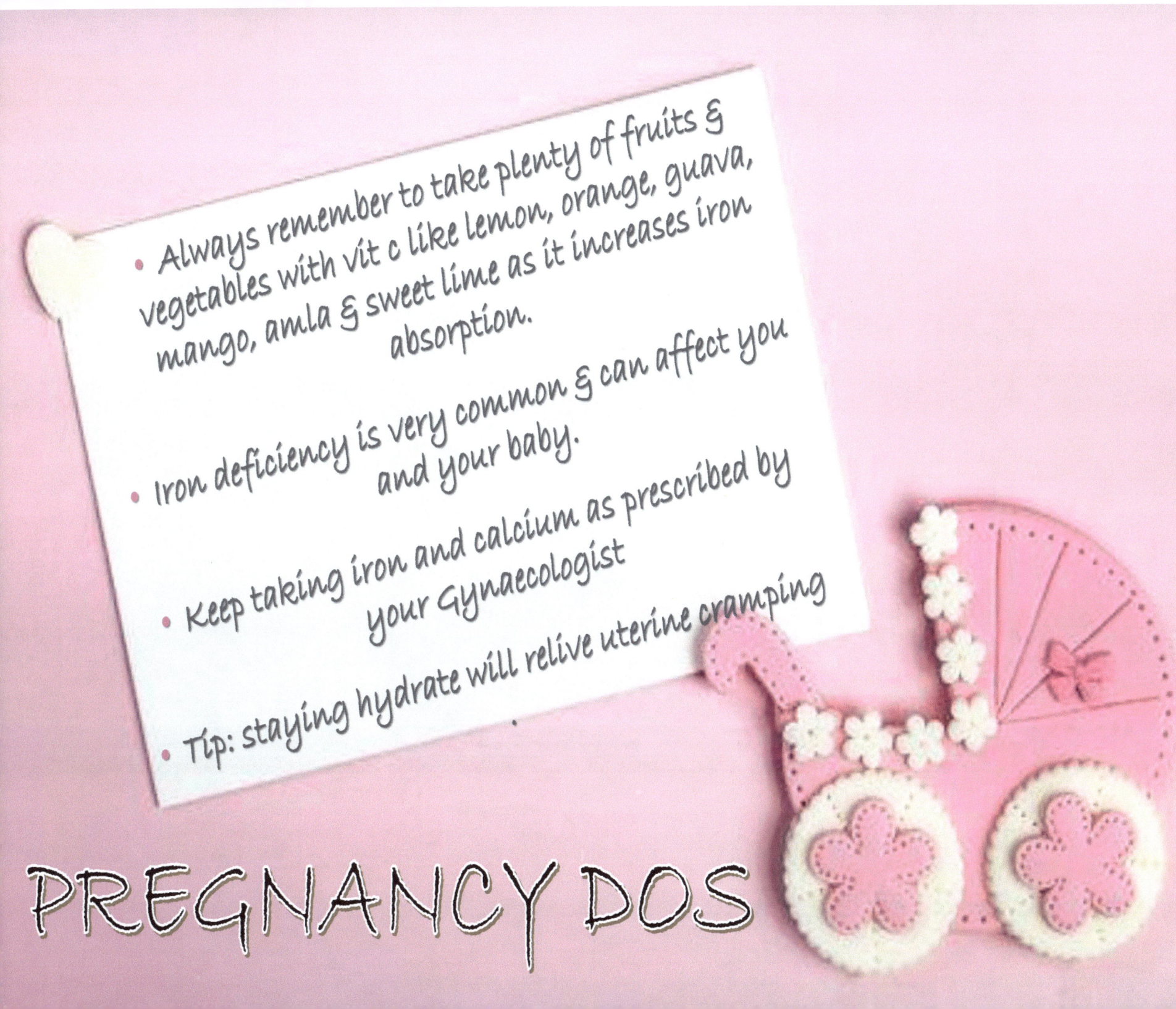

PREGNANCY DOS

- Always remember to take plenty of fruits & vegetables with vit c like lemon, orange, guava, mango, amla & sweet lime as it increases iron absorption.
- Iron deficiency is very common & can affect you and your baby.
- Keep taking iron and calcium as prescribed by your Gynaecologist
- Tip: staying hydrate will relive uterine cramping

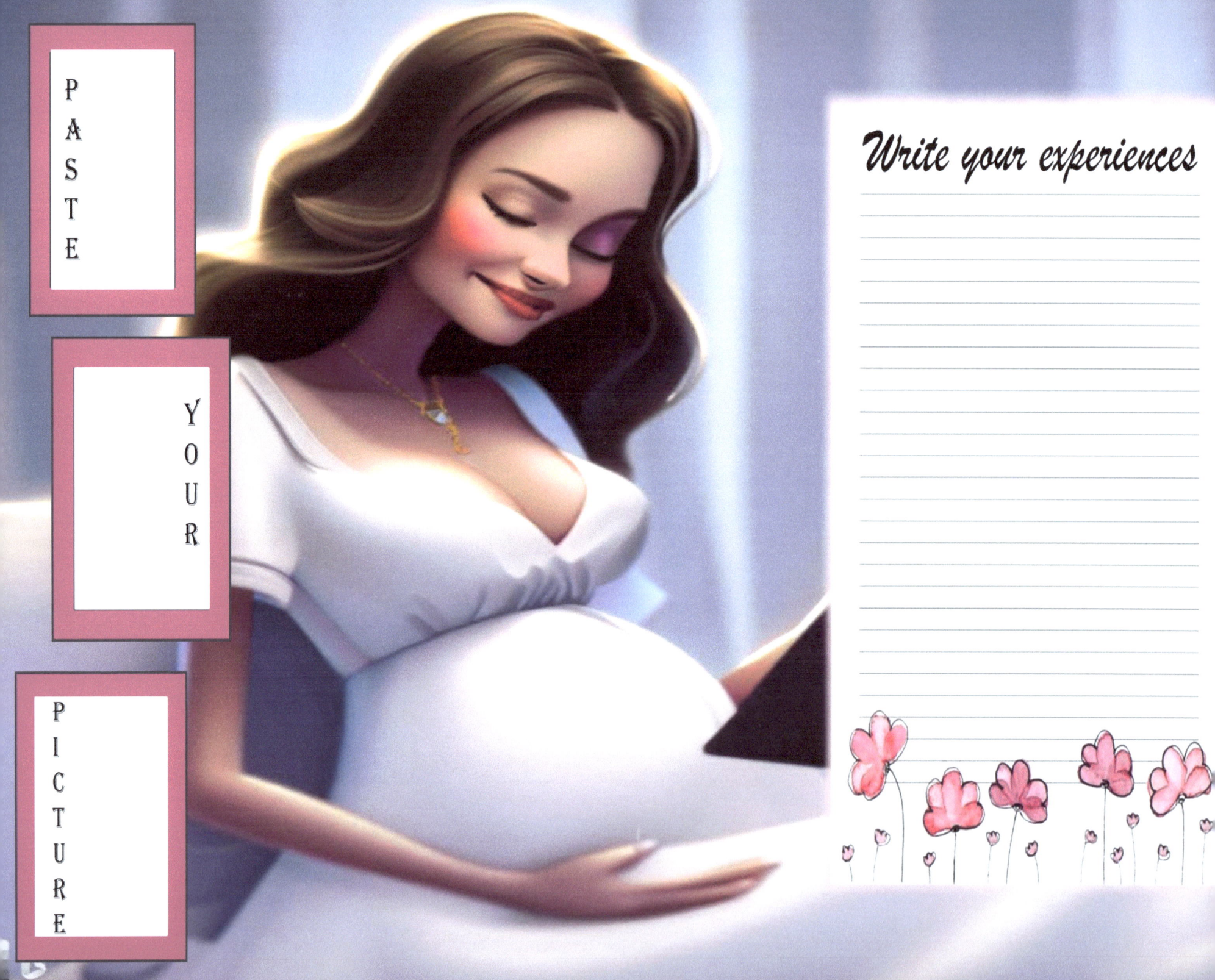

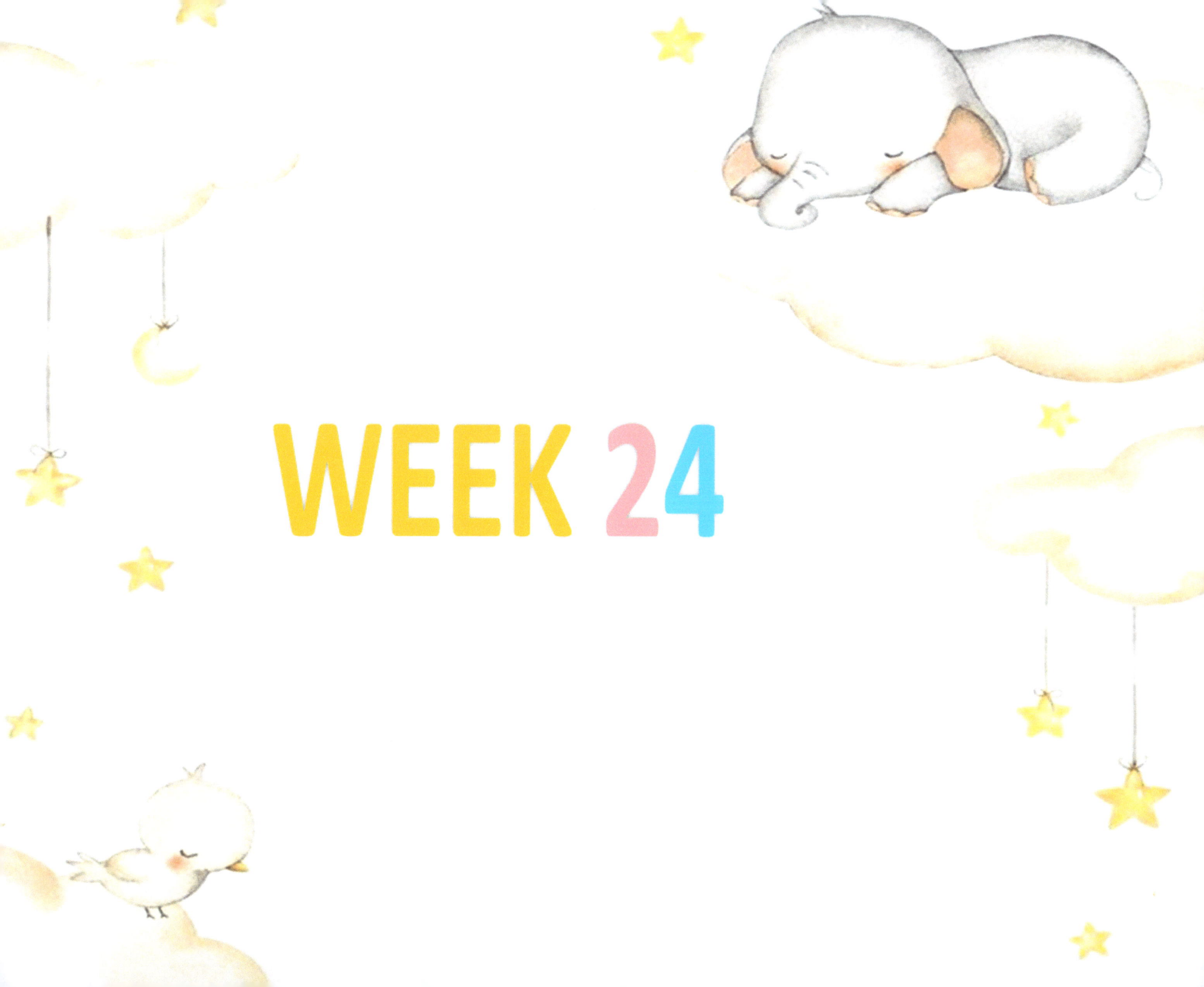

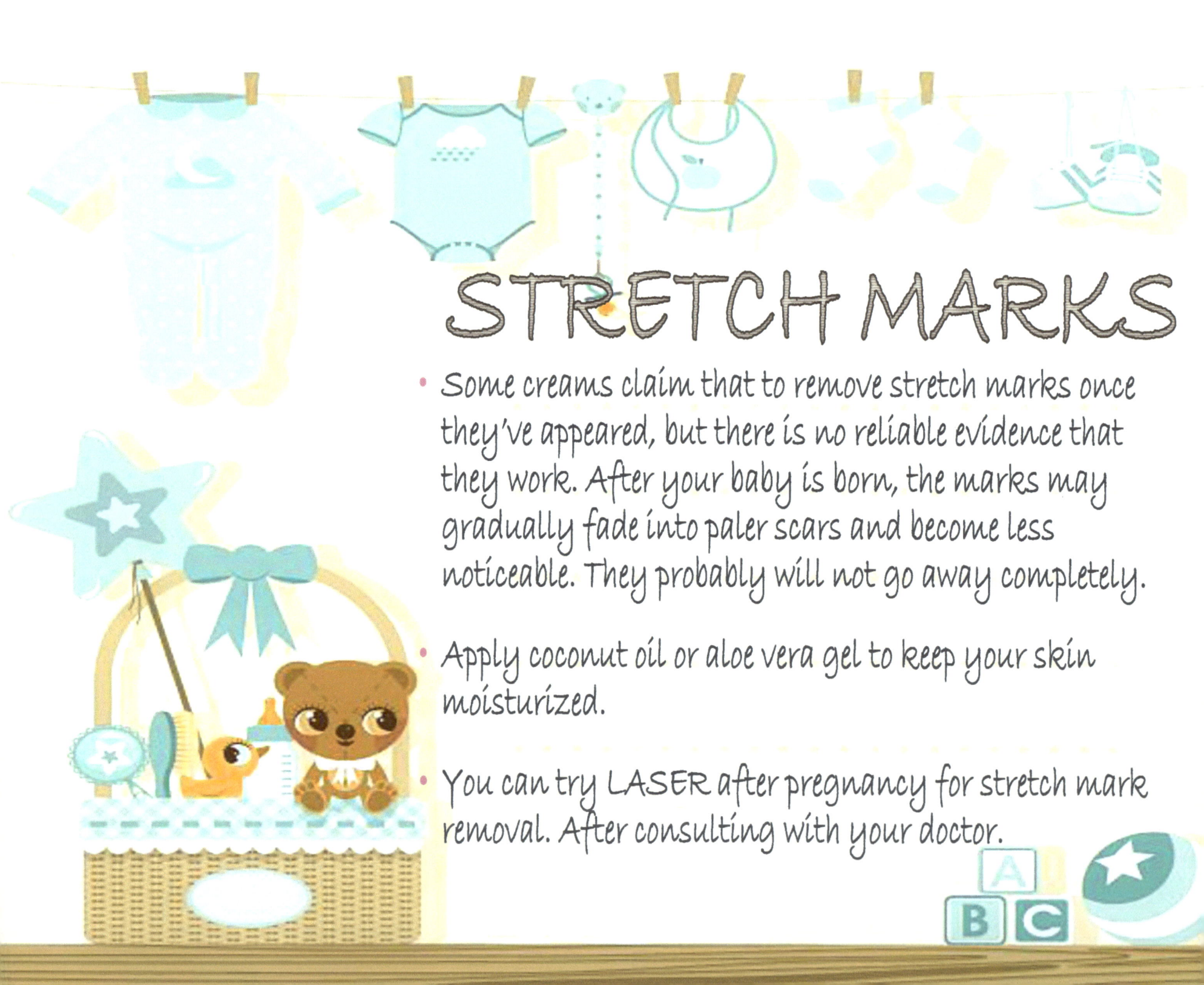

HIGH BLOOD PRESSURE DURING PREGNANCY

HYPERTENSION IN PREGNANCY

SYSTOLIC BLOOD PRESSURE >= 140 mmHg or
DIASTOLIC BLOOD PRESSURE >= 90 mmHg

ACOG 2023

High blood pressure may causes several issues to the baby during pregnancy. To avoid this, the sodium-potassium balance must be maintained.

- High sodium increases risk of high blood pressure. Increase potassium rich foods like fresh guava, kiwi, banana, pomegranate, cherries, litchis etc.

- **TIP: Have a banana everyday.**

EXERCISE IN PREGNANCY

Weeks 25-28

Continue with low-impact cardio exercises, focusing on activities that are gentle on the joints, such as stationary cycling or water aerobics. Modify exercises as your belly grows to ensure comfort and safety. Incorporate exercises that strengthen the core muscles, such as modified planks or seated exercises.

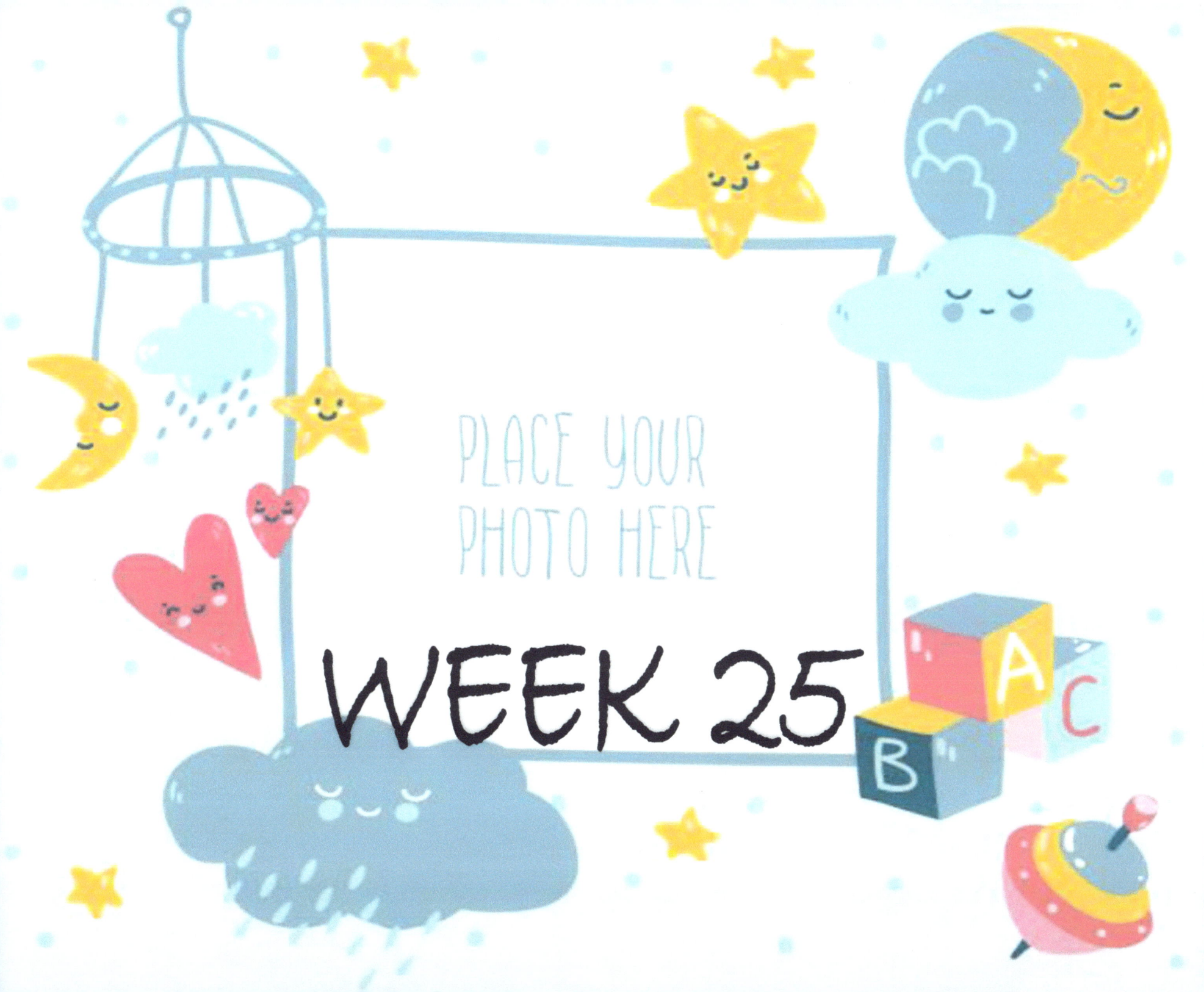
WEEK 25

KNOW YOUR BABY

- **Your baby can hear you!** Their hearing is developing quickly and, at 25 weeks pregnant, she may even start to respond to familiar sounds like your voice by moving or changing her position. Give it a try!

- Here comes the concept of Garbhsanskar

- Tip: involve your partner while talking with the baby, this will help baby to bond easily with the father.

SKIN CHANGES IN PREGNANCY

- Hormonal changes taking place in pregnancy may your nipples and the area around them go darker. Your skin color may also darken a little, either in patches or all over.

- Birthmarks, moles and freckles may also darken. You may develop a dark line down the middle of your stomach. These changes will gradually fade after the baby is born, although your nipples may remain a little darker.

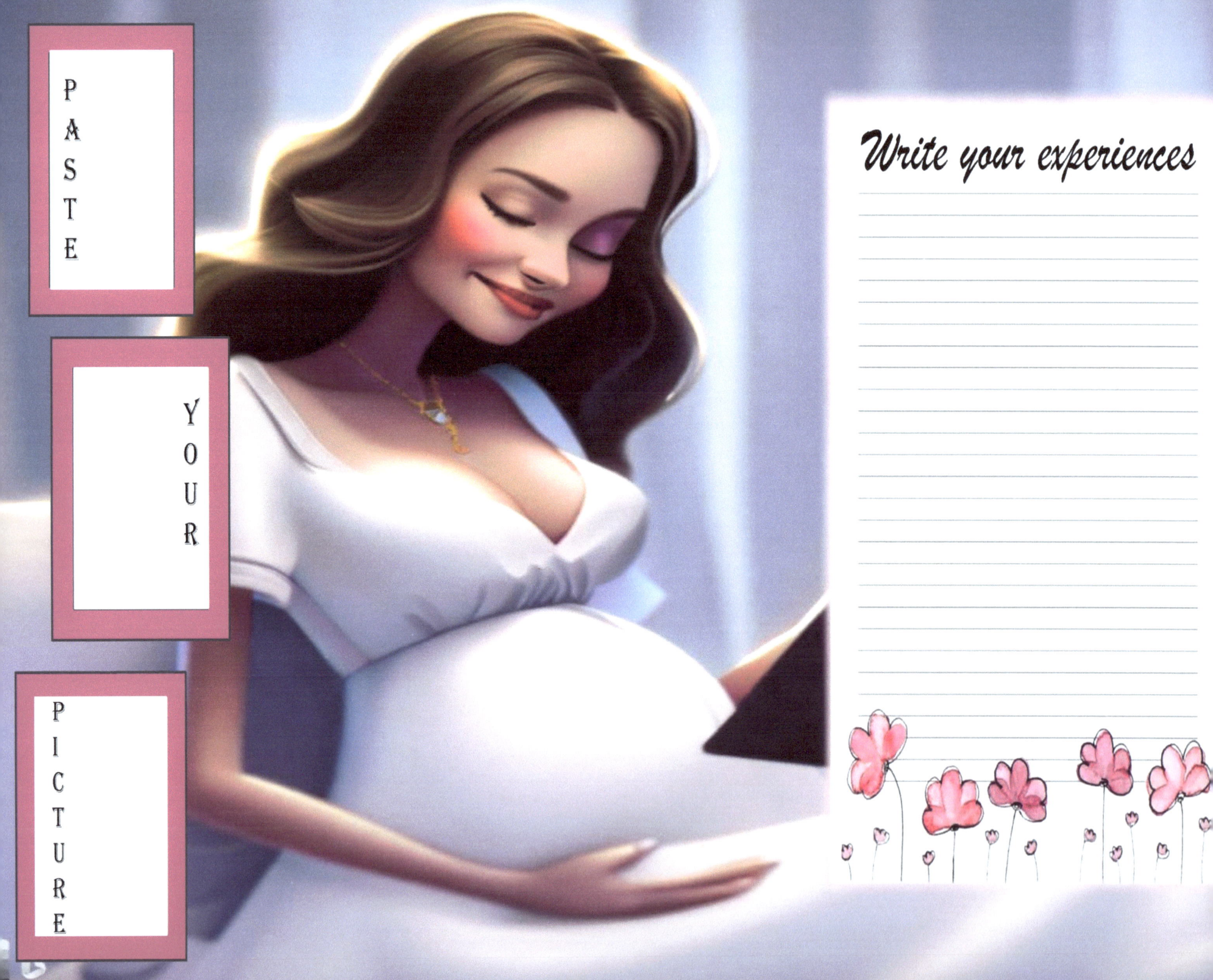

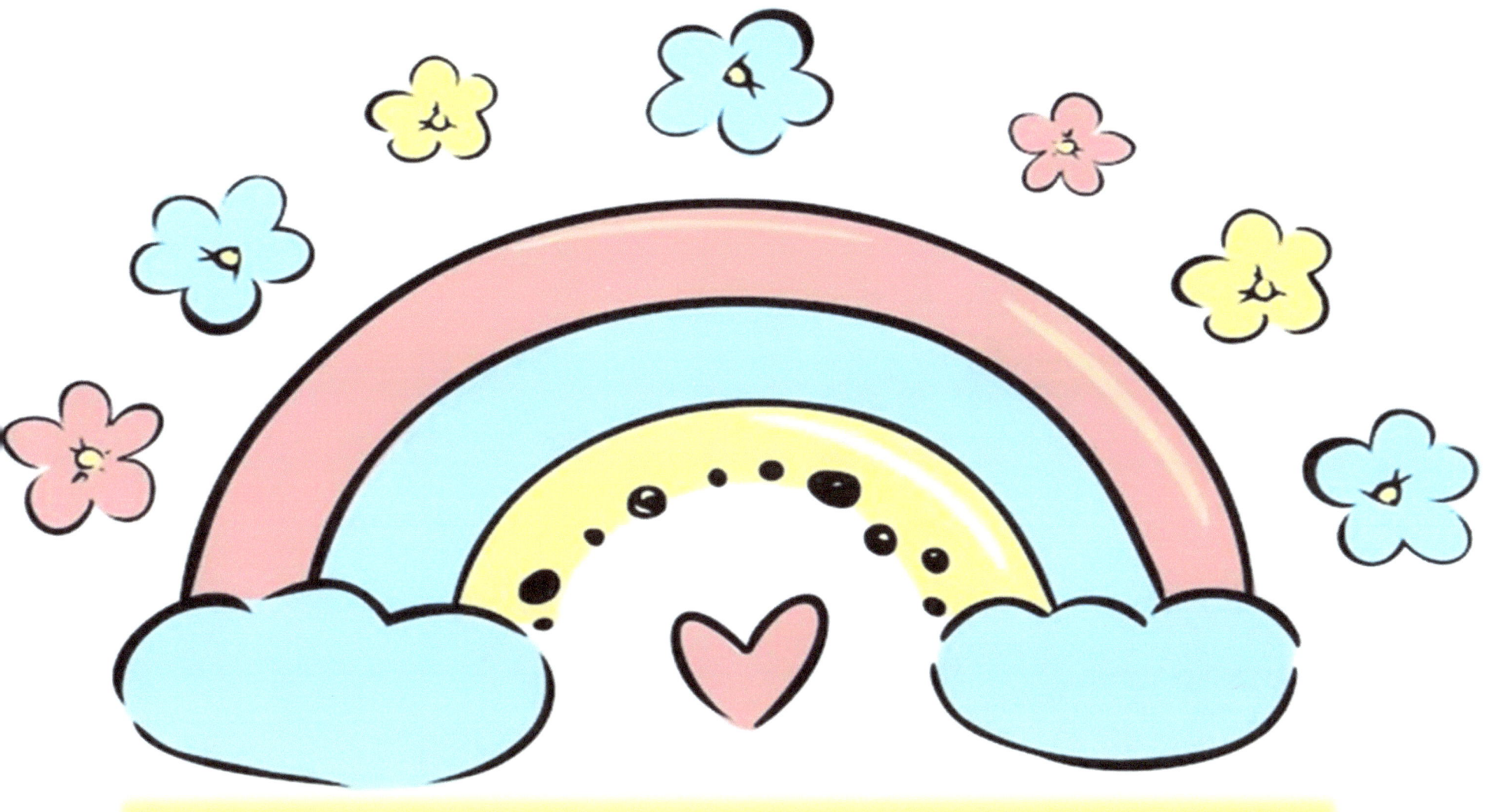

HAVING A URINE INFECTION

- During pregnancy, it's a quite common to have urine infection Keep your genital area clean & dry to prevent this.

- If you have pain during passing urine, fever or a strong feeling to pass urine every time, contact the doctor to check for any chances of infection

Balanced Diet

Fat deposition is at peak, so proper nutrition and balanced diet is very important around this week. Follow a healthy diet plan to keep your weight in check.

KNOW YOUR BABY

- At this time your baby's lung is growing. Also, he/she can suck their thumb fingers inside the womb. Interesting right?

- Soon your baby will open their eyes & start blinking in a few weeks.

- Listening to calming music is proven to improve brain development in baby

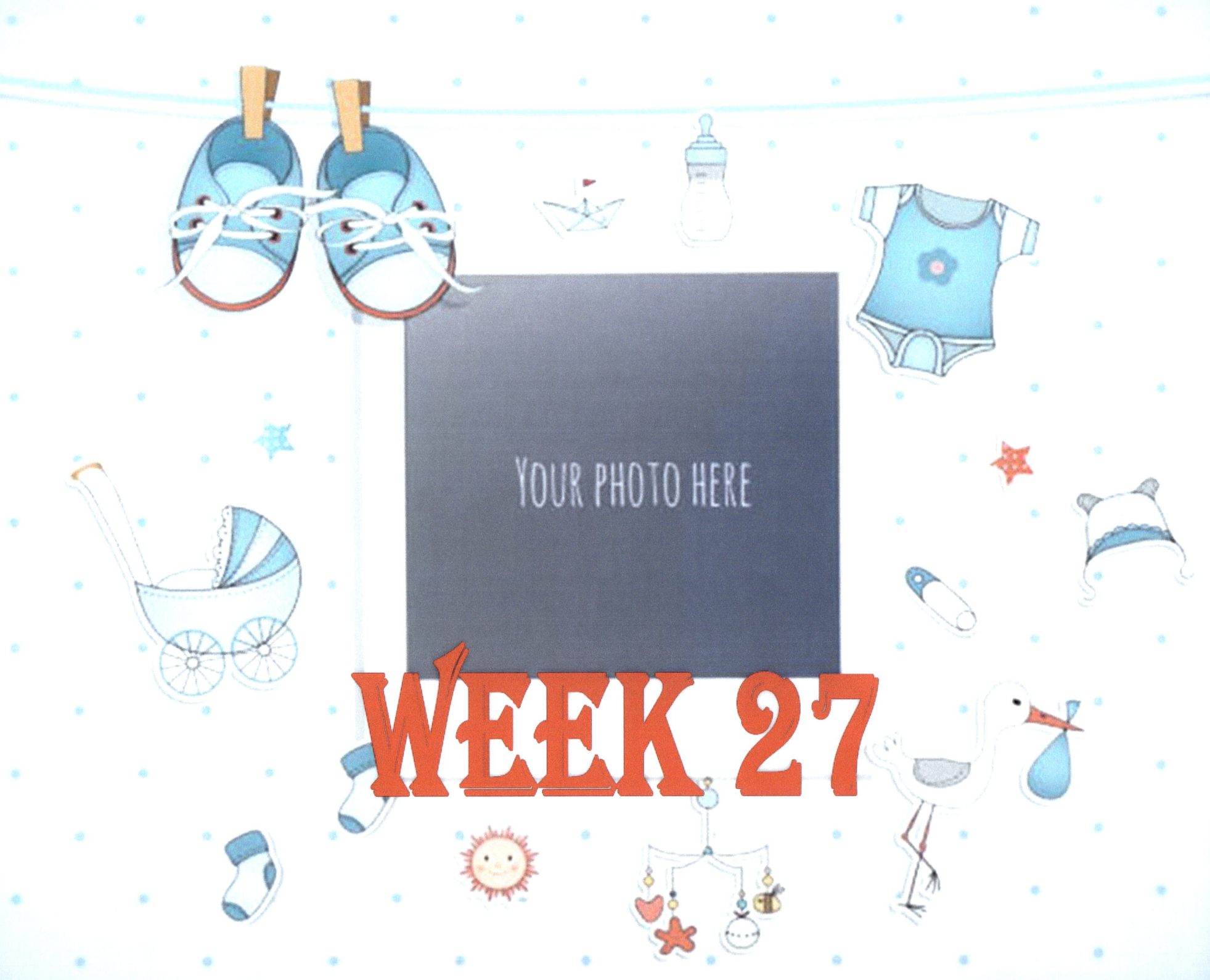

FACING PIGMENTATION ON SKIN

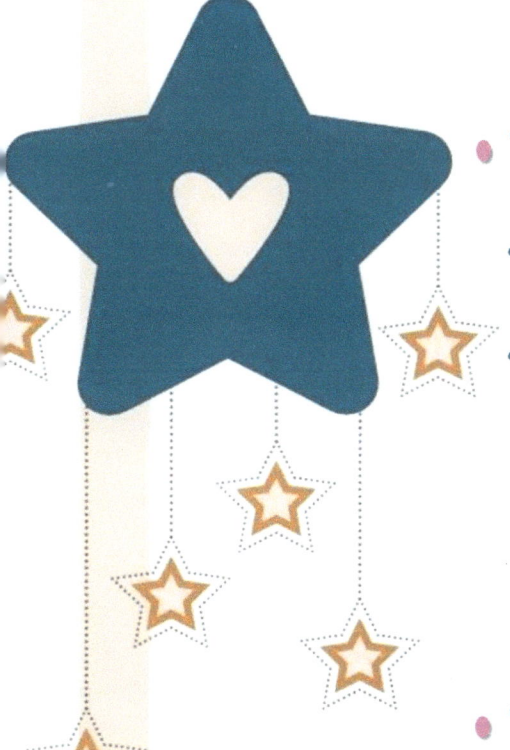

- Pregnancy hormones can cause hyper pigmentation of the skin. This can result in pronounced freckles or moles, a dark line down or brown patches on cheeks called melasma.

- Don't worry, most pigmentation fade in few months after giving birth when your body starts to recover.

TALK TO YOUR BABY

- Your baby has started to kick now, also he/she can recognize voices around you. And you know what's special, your baby's heart rate slows down when she/he hears your voice. Which means he/she is calm and relaxed.

- Talk to your baby regularly. You may feel the fetal movements all prominent around the time.

PASTE

YOUR

PICTURE

Write your experiences

HAIR CARE IN PREGNANCY

Third Trimester

Scalp and Hair Hygiene: Maintain good scalp hygiene by regularly washing your hair and keeping it clean. This can help prevent any buildup or irritation.

Gentle Hair Care: Be extra gentle when brushing or styling your hair to minimize breakage. Use a wide-toothed comb or a brush with soft bristles to avoid pulling or tugging.

Hair Accessories: Opt for loose hairstyles and avoid tight ponytails or braids that can put strain on your hair. Use soft, fabric-covered hair ties to prevent breakage

SKIN CARE IN PREGNANCY

Third Trimester

Intense Hydration: As your skin stretches further, it may become drier. Increase your moisturizing routine and consider using a thicker cream or oil to provide intense hydration.

Soothing Irritation: If you experience itching or skin irritation, consult your healthcare provider to rule out any underlying conditions. They may recommend pregnancy-safe creams or ointments to alleviate discomfort.

Avoid Harsh Chemicals: Be cautious of skincare products containing potentially harmful ingredients such as retinoids, hydroquinone, or high concentrations of essential oils. Stick to gentle, natural ingredients to minimize the risk of adverse effects on your baby.

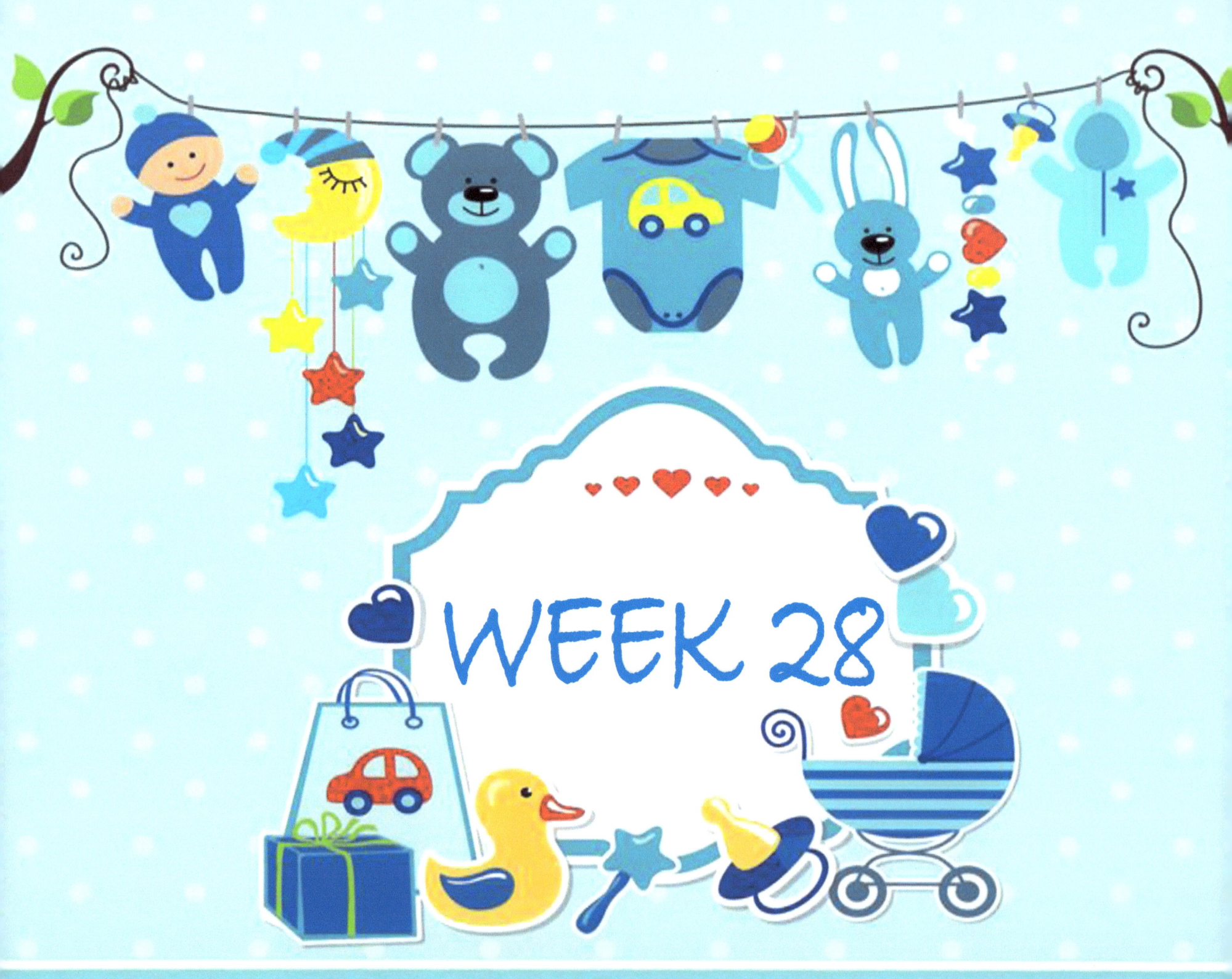

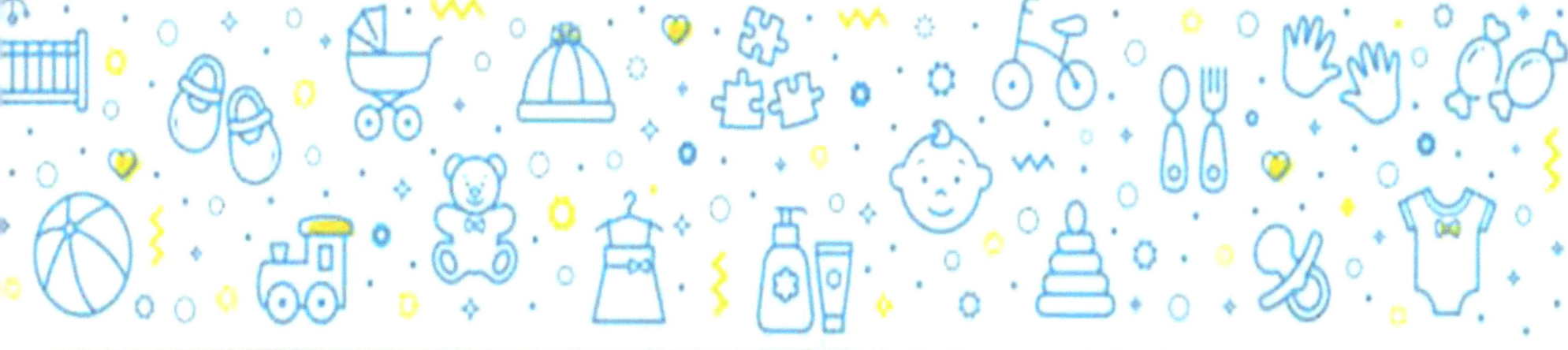

ARE YOU DOING DAILY KICKS COUNTS?

- Your baby must be moving or kicking inside the womb. It is common during this time of pregnancy.

- Three counts each of 1 hour duration (morning, afternoon and evening) are recommended. The total counts multiplied by 4 gives DFMC (daily fetal movement count) If it is less it indicates warning sign. visit your doctor.

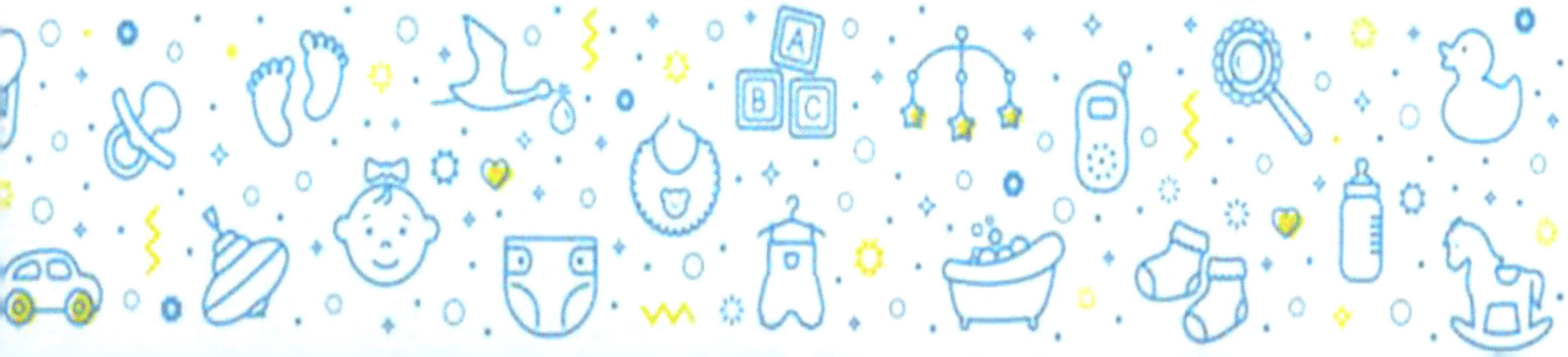

EXERCISE IN PREGNANCY

Weeks 29-32

Engage in exercises that promote good posture, such as prenatal yoga or Pilates. Include exercises that strengthen the legs and prepare for labor, such as squats or prenatal strength training with light weights. Avoid exercises that involve lying flat on your back to prevent supine hypotensive syndrome.

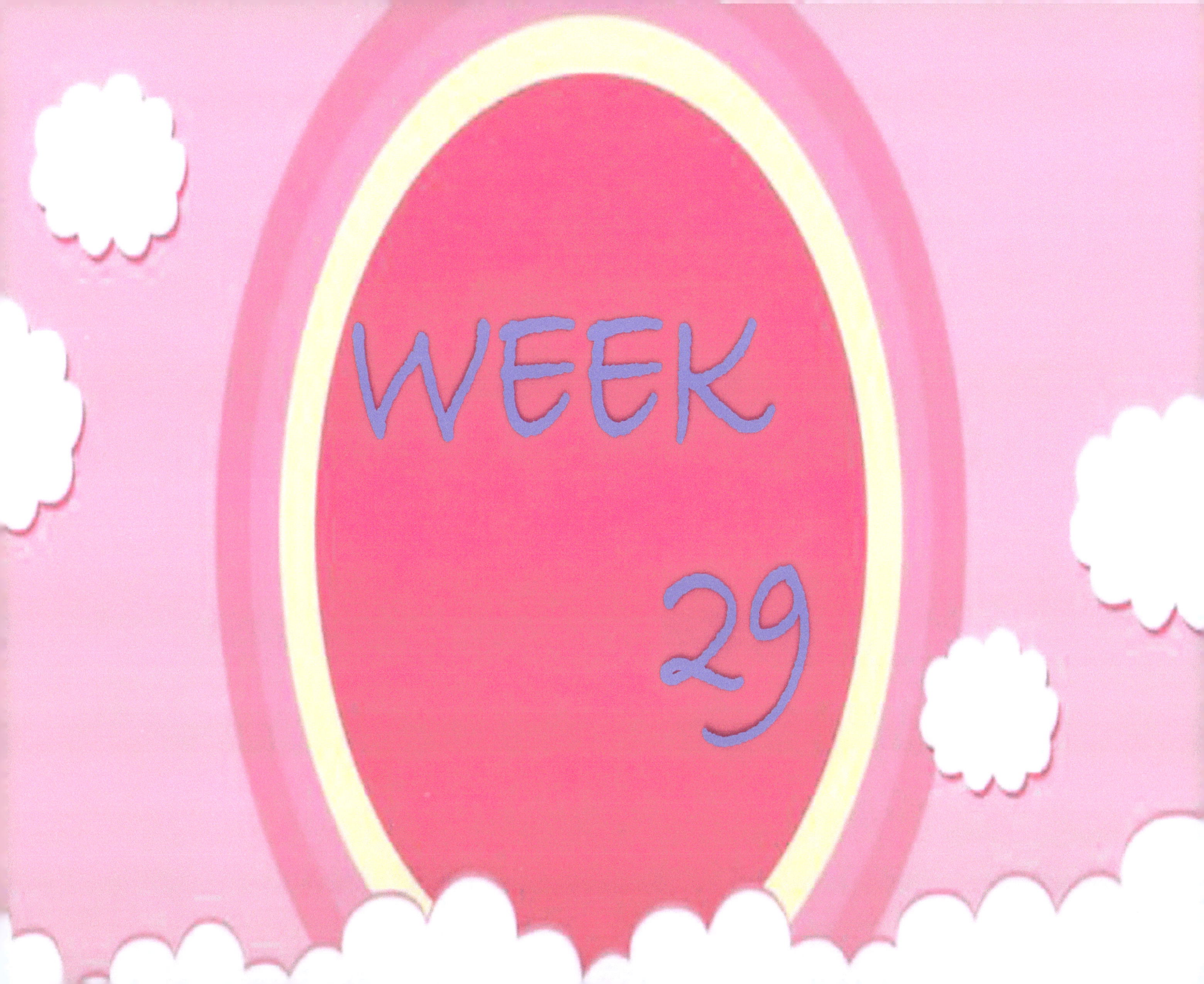

SLEEP PROBLEMS

- Leg cramps, acidity, frequent visit of bathroom & anxiety during theses weeks along with hormonal changes can lead to sleep problems. To handle anxiety, frequently talk to our partner, family & friends to stay distressed.

- You can discuss it with your doctor and consult a psychiatrist if you feel too anxious. meditation and exercise will surely help you tackle insomnia.

CHANGE IN FETAL MOVEMENT

- You may experience more activity of your baby in the coming weeks of pregnancy. Especially after your meals & while you are lying down. You might feel hard kicks too. But don't worry, keep in touch with your gynecologist about any changes in the movement.

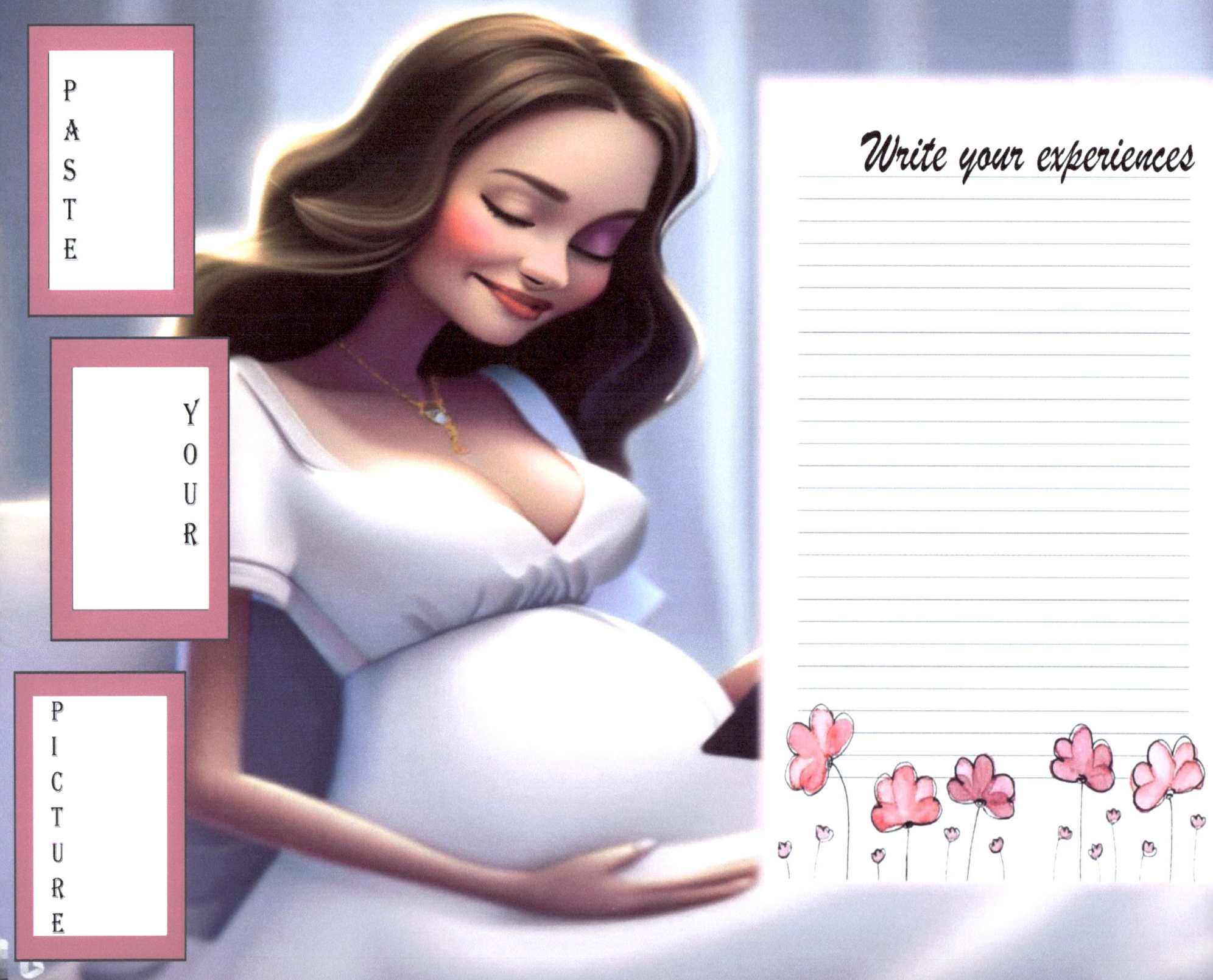

WEEK 30

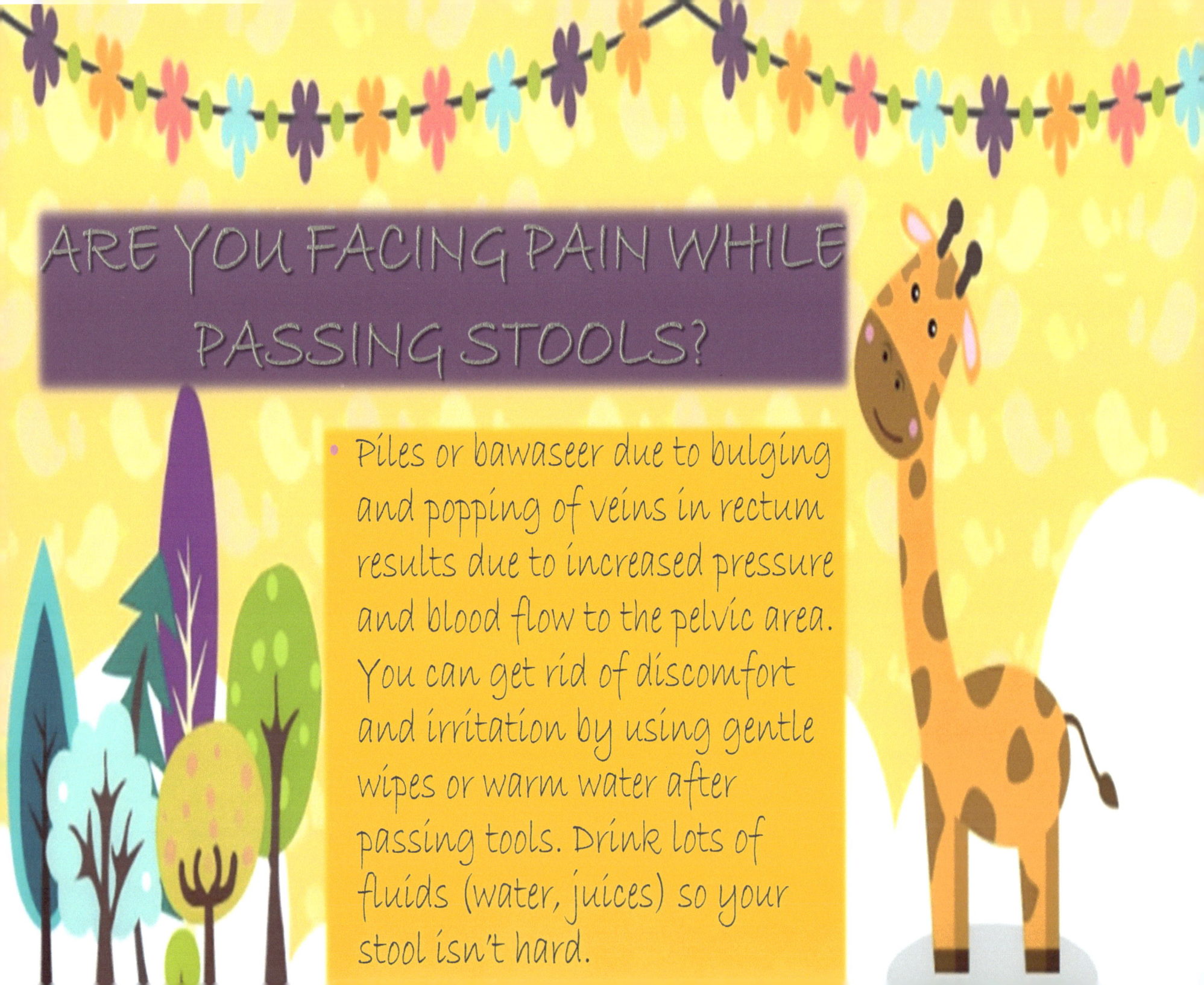

ARE YOU FACING PAIN WHILE PASSING STOOLS?

- Piles or bawaseer due to bulging and popping of veins in rectum results due to increased pressure and blood flow to the pelvic area. You can get rid of discomfort and irritation by using gentle wipes or warm water after passing tools. Drink lots of fluids (water, juices) so your stool isn't hard.

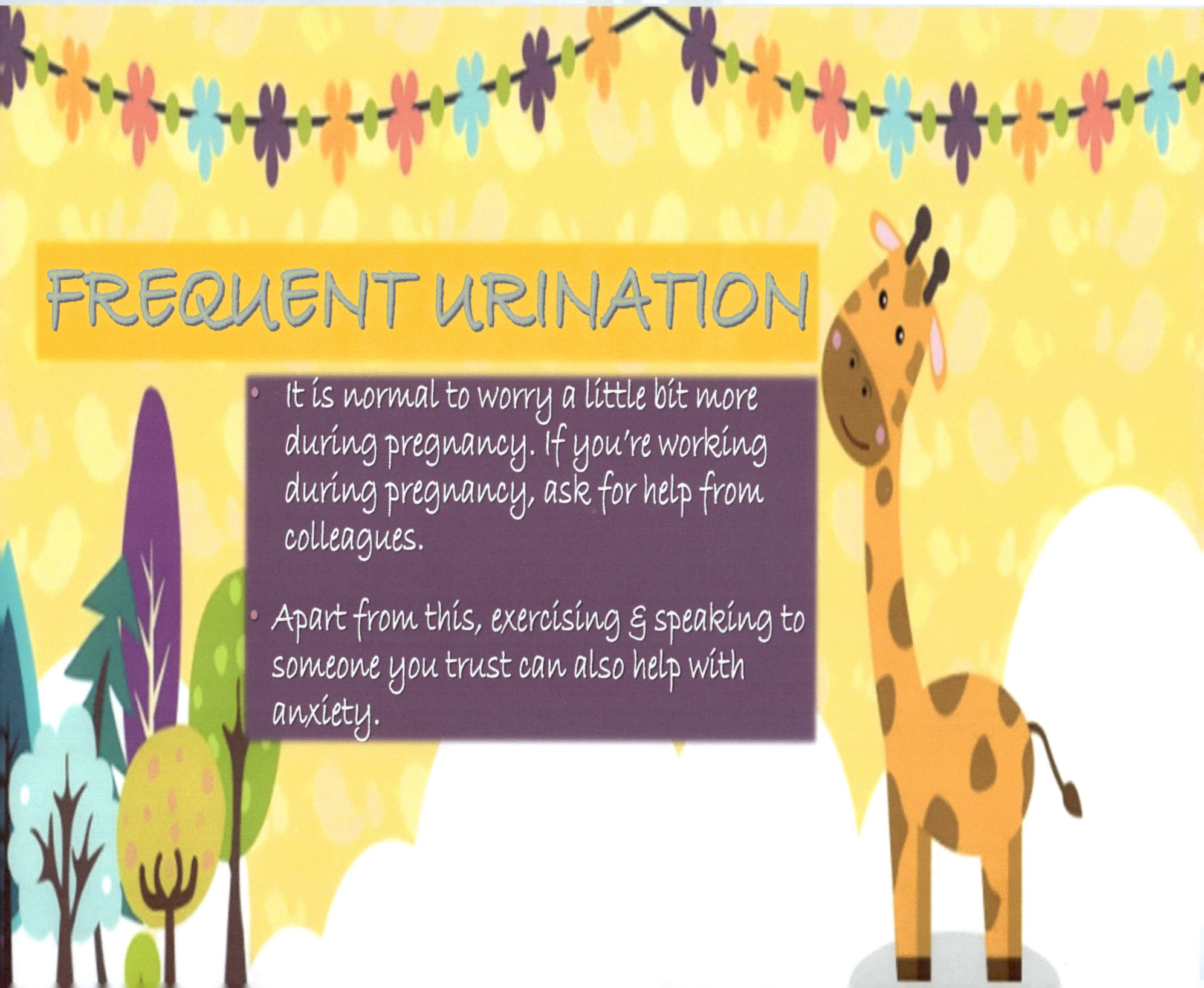

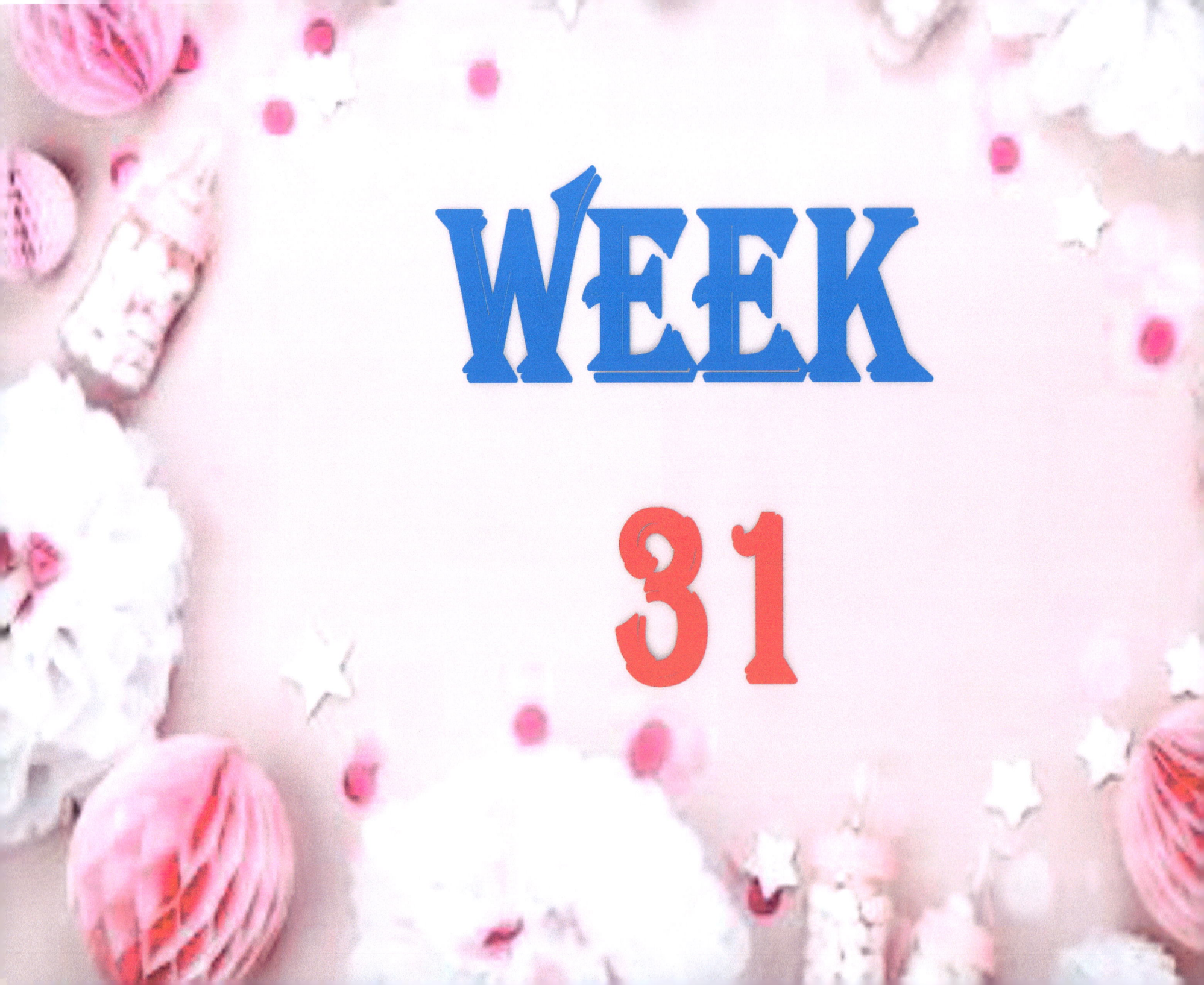

MILKY DISCHARGE FROM BREASTS

- As your breasts get bigger, they may also leak a yellowish fluid called colostrum, which is the precursor to breast milk. This liquid packed with protein and antibodies, is the first milk your baby will get. If the leaks are getting uncomfortable, try wearing nursing pads for breast support.

- Wearing a good bra is essential so that the breasts don't sag later on.

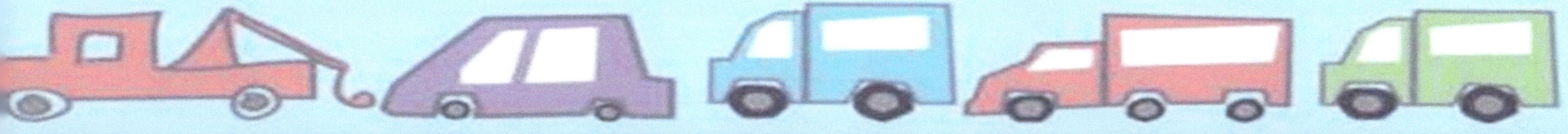

ARE BABY MOVEMENTS DISCOMFORTING?

- We completely understand that it can be uncomfortable that to be bear those baby kicks. But it is also a sign that your baby is active & healthy, so take it positively.

- Keep tracking fetal kicks counts.

HAVE LIGHT MEALS AT NIGHT

- Have light meals at night. This could be vegetables soups, fruit salad, raita with dahi, green leafy vegetables or roti. Don't strain excessively while on the toilet (constipation-related straining can actually cause piles).

- Drink plenty of water to keep your digestive tract active.

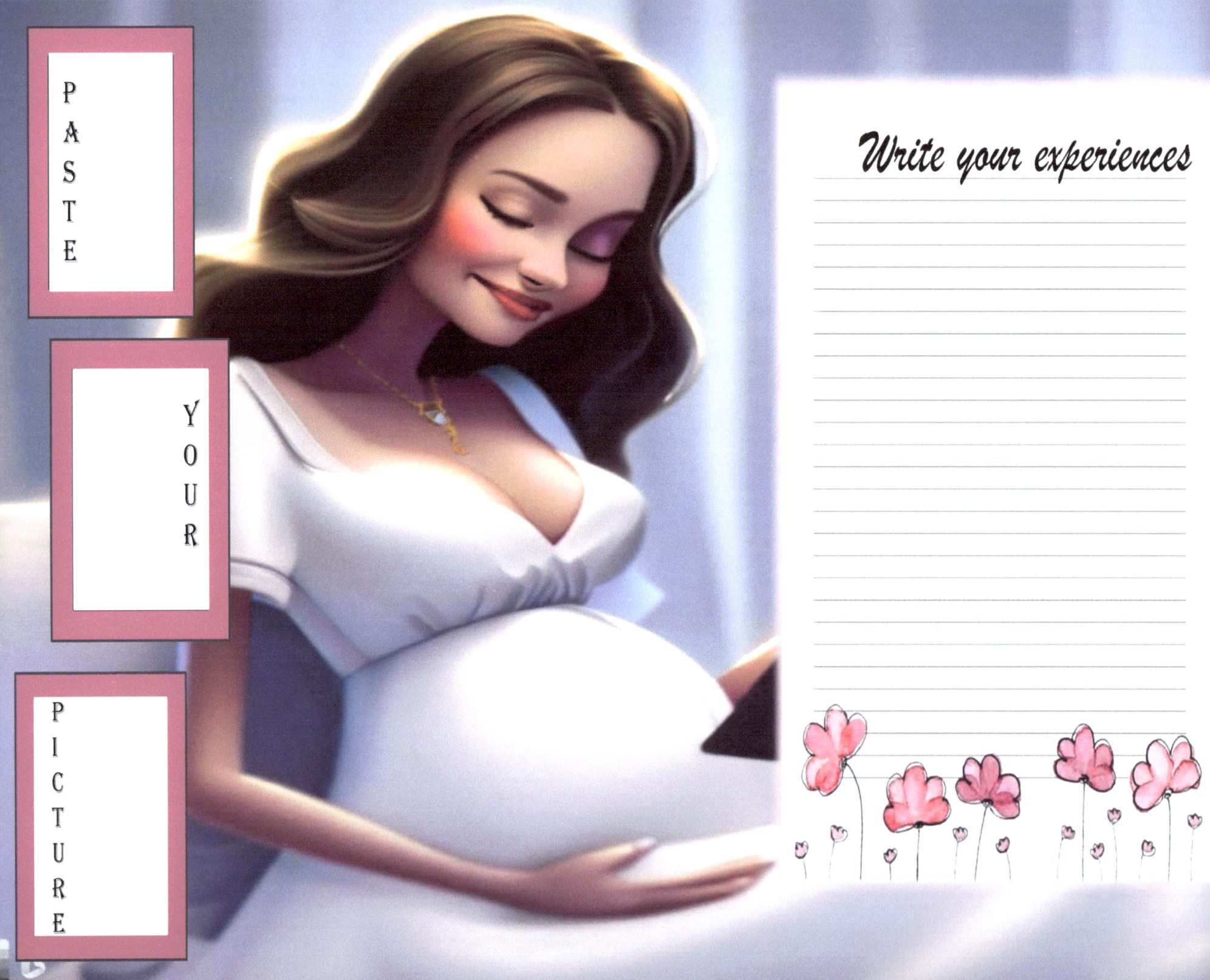

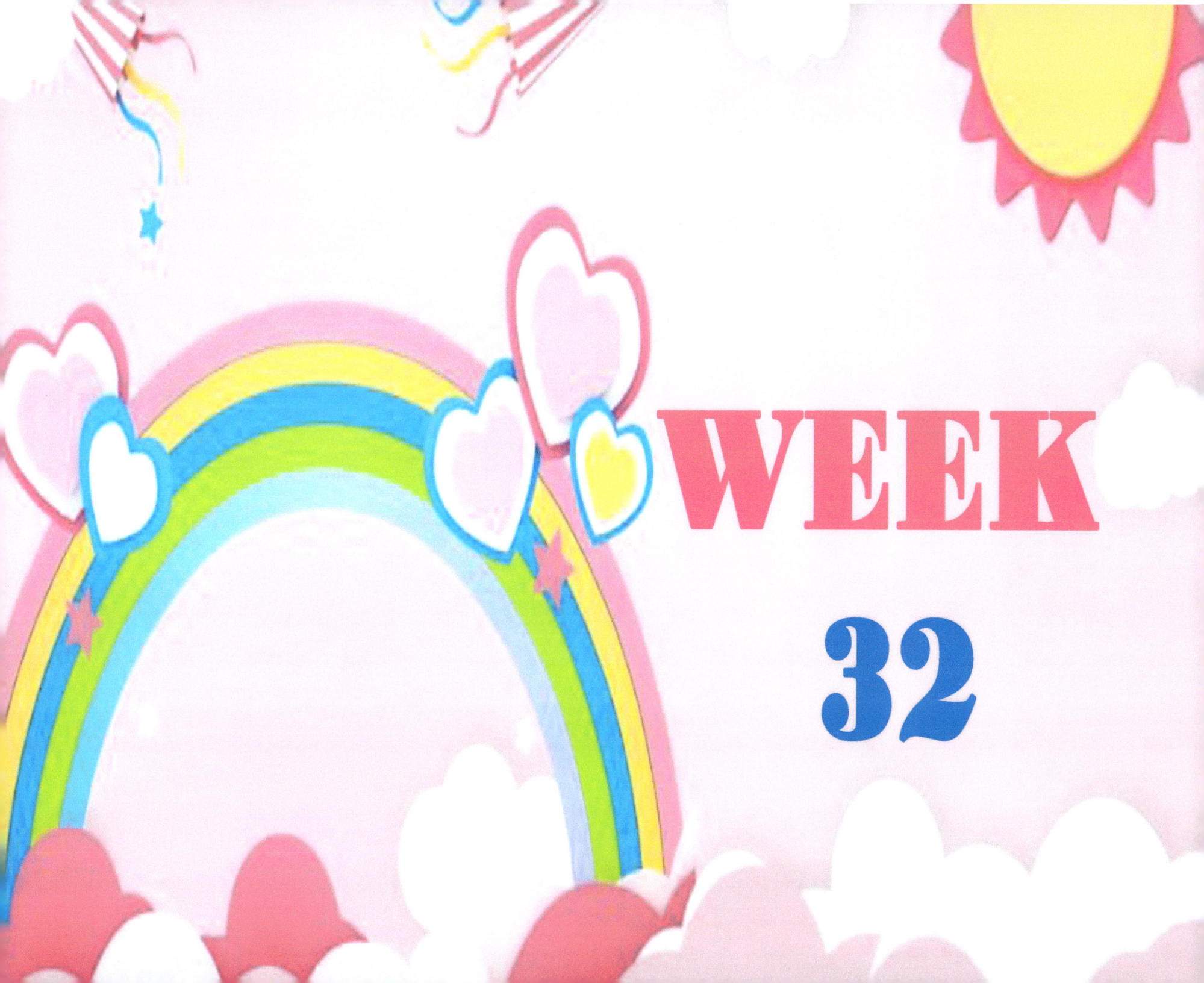

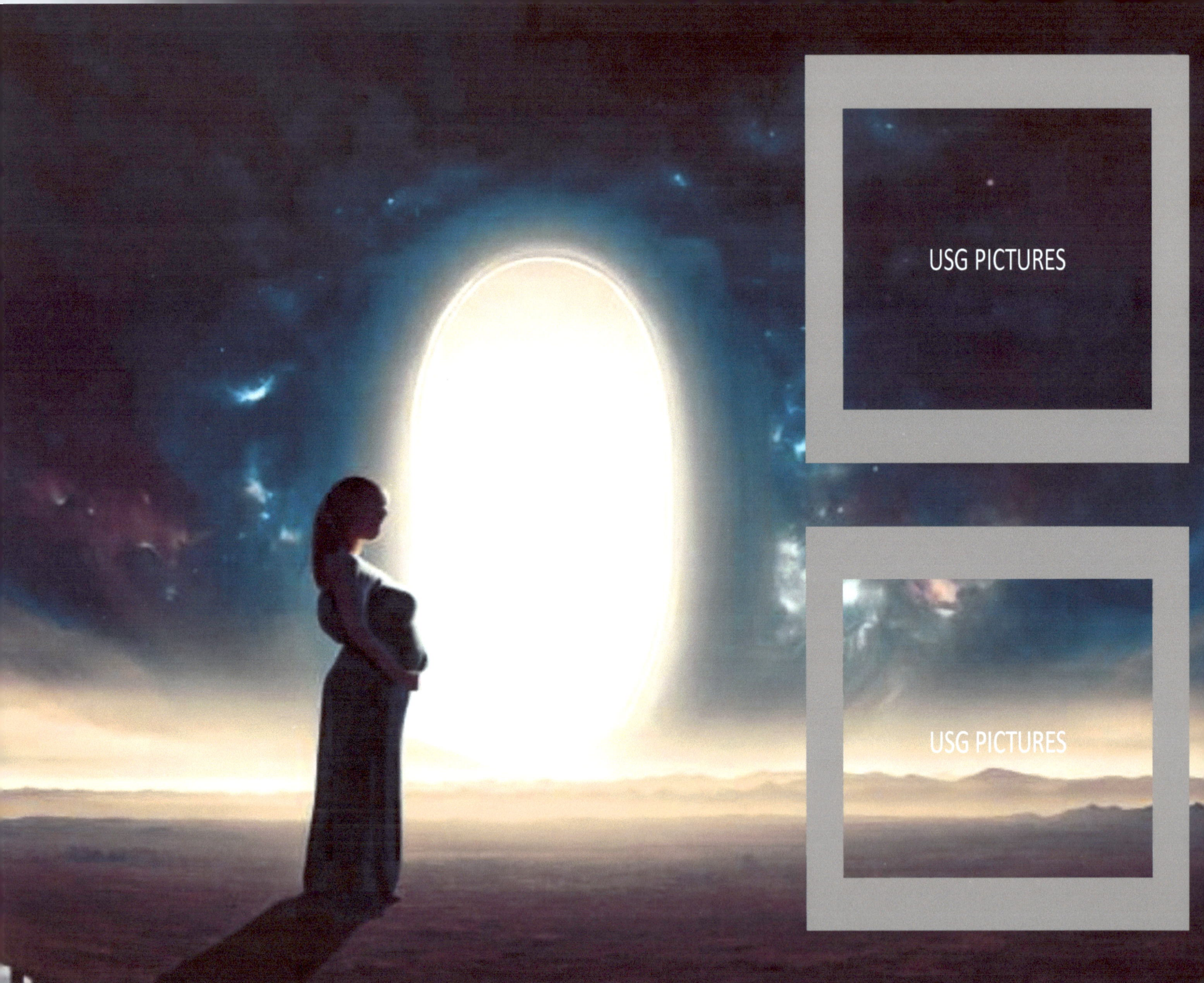

BEWARE OF FALSE CONTRACTIONS

- These practice contractions are most often felt by moms who've already gone through a pregnancy.

- How do you know they're not the real thing? Even at their most intense, changing your position from sitting to lying down, from lying down to walking around, will usually make them disappear.

Pregnancy DONT's

- Do not wear tight fitting clothes as it can be uncomfortable & put undue pressure on the womb. Your shoes should also be comfortable.

- Tip: Continue with pelvic floor exercises and breathing to prepare your body for the labour day.

EXERCISE IN PREGNANCY

Weeks 33-36

Focus on exercises that help maintain flexibility and prepare for childbirth, such as prenatal yoga or gentle stretching. Continue with low-impact cardio activities, but be mindful of your body's limits. Consider pelvic tilts and hip circles to alleviate any pelvic discomfort.

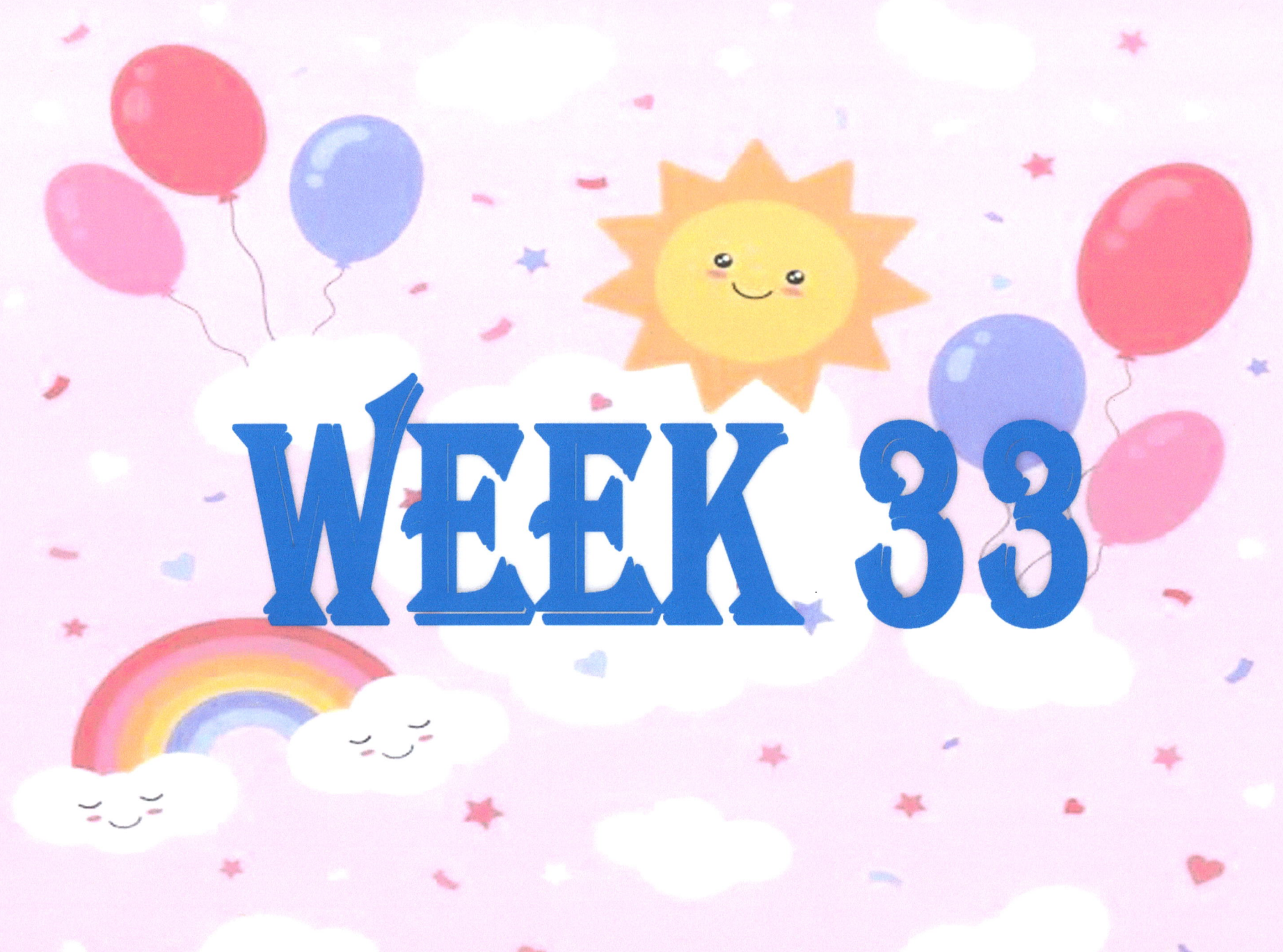

FIND MORE ABOUT BREASTFEEDING

- it is the perfect time to read & understand more about breastfeeding.

- A newborn child should only be given breast milk. There is a lot of false information about breast feeding on the internet. Talk to your doctor if you have any doubts.

PREGNANCY DO'S

- Keep in mind that in the coming 7 weeks, you will undergo labour. Labour may be painful & it is very important to be physically, mentally & emotionally ready for this experience. This is very natural. You can share your anxiety with your doctor.

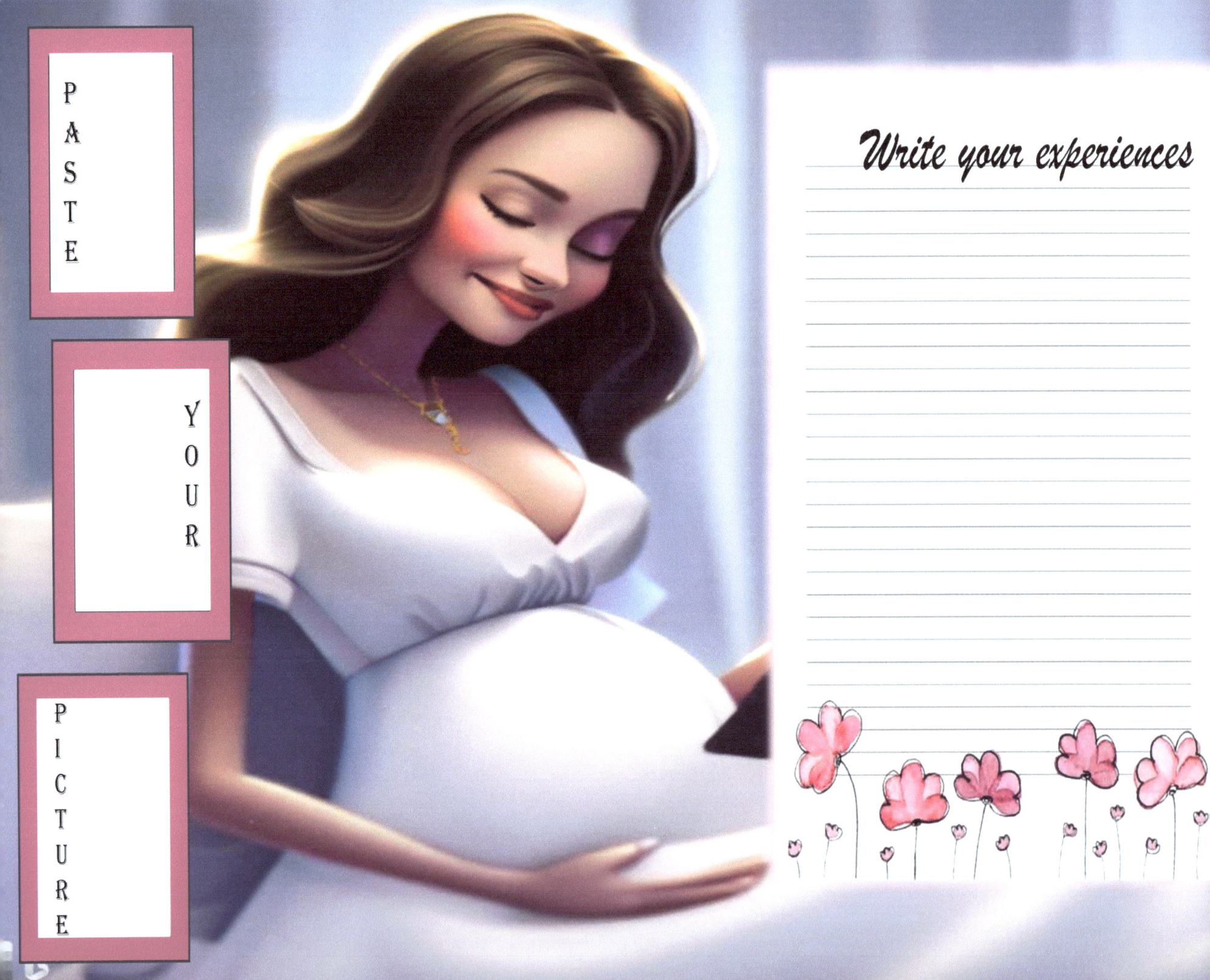

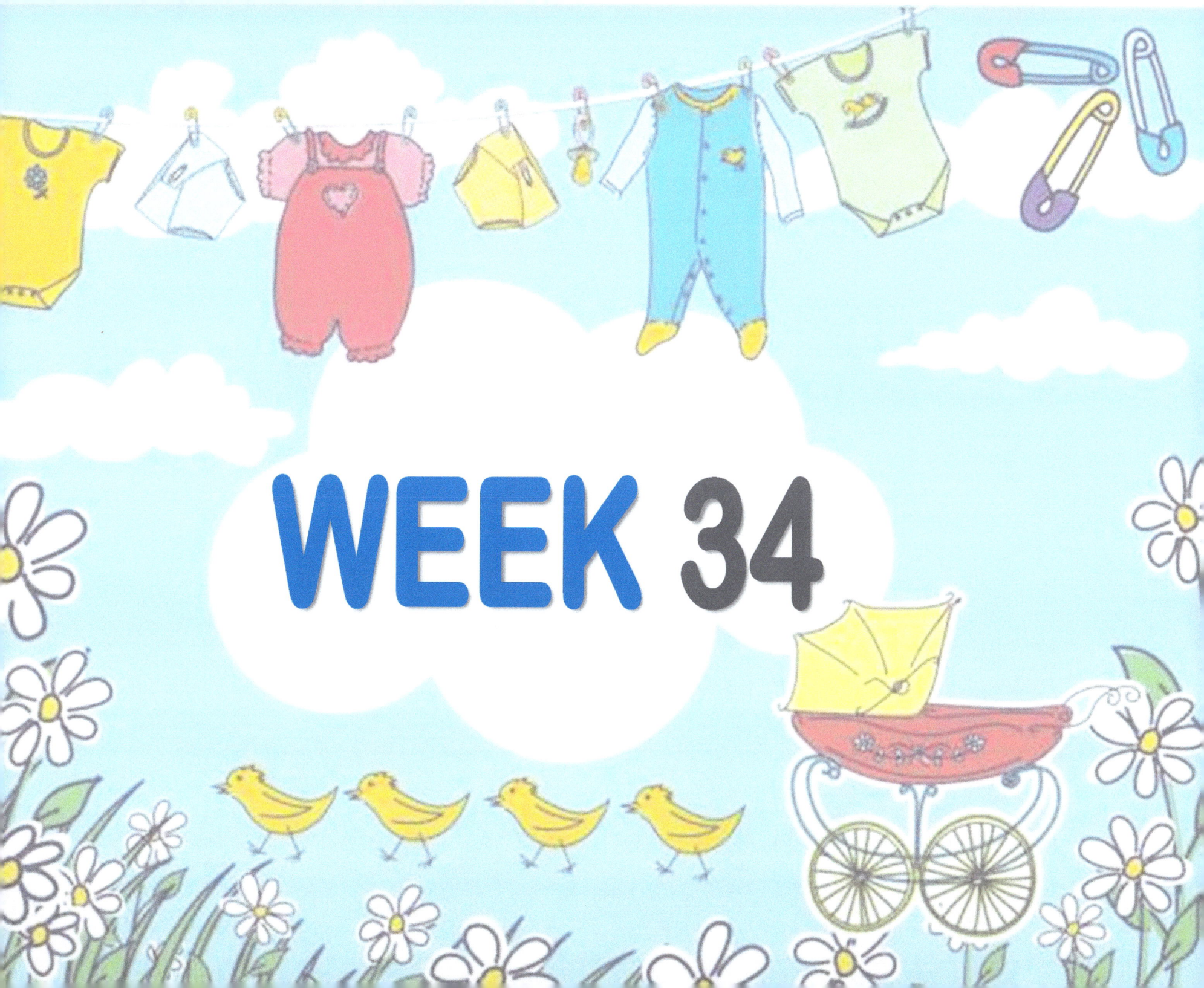

We can't wait to meet you
BABY

KEEP YOUR BAGS READY!

- Grip socks
- Basic toiletries
- Hospital Gowns
- Pillow and blankets
- Thick sanitary pads
- Large cup for water and ice
- Disposable mesh underwater
- Labor tools, like personal massagers
- After care items like watch, hazel pads and peri bottles.

CONSTIPATION

- It will be difficult to clear your bowels. Apart from gentle exercise, you can consume lots of water to keep your motions clear.

- Also, please have high fiber foods like fresh fruits, green leafy vegetables, salads, whole grain bread (not brown or white bread). eat smaller meals in place of heavy ones.

Do you have following symptoms?

Please report such symptoms to your doctor.

- Soreness of palms and soles
- Itching that get worse at night
- Dark Urine
- Pale or grey bowel movements
- Right-sided upper abdominal pain.

Pregnancy DONTs

- Do not panic when you experience labour. Labour is a natural process during childbirth. Always make sure that you are not alone during this time.

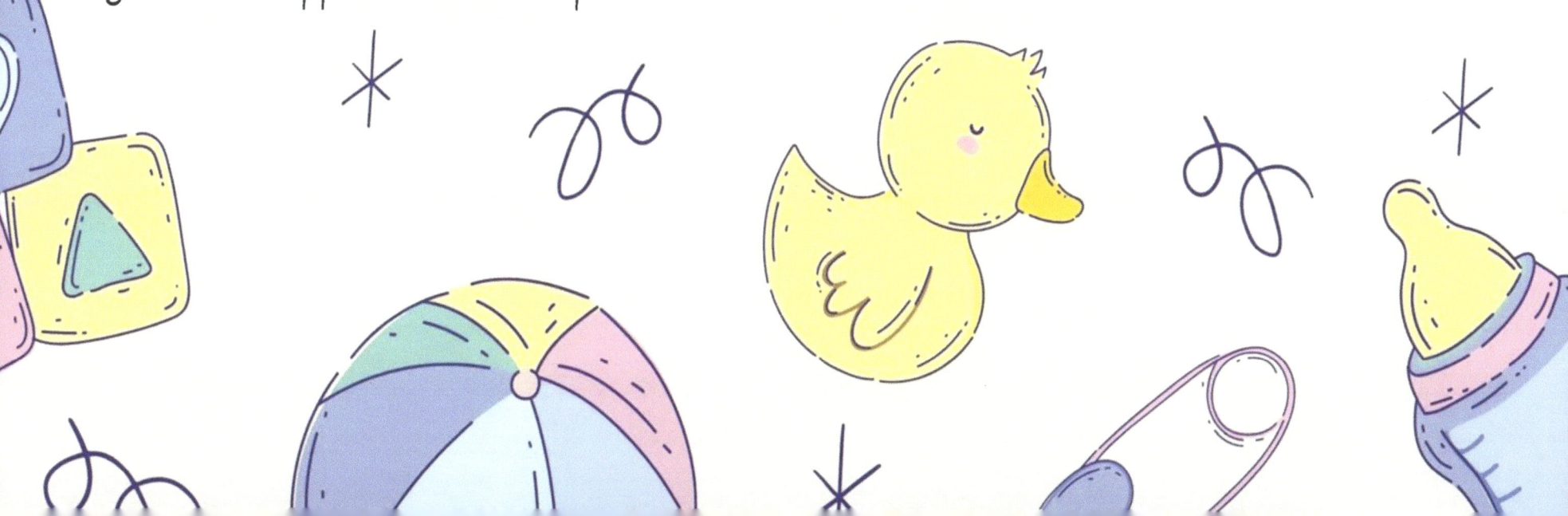

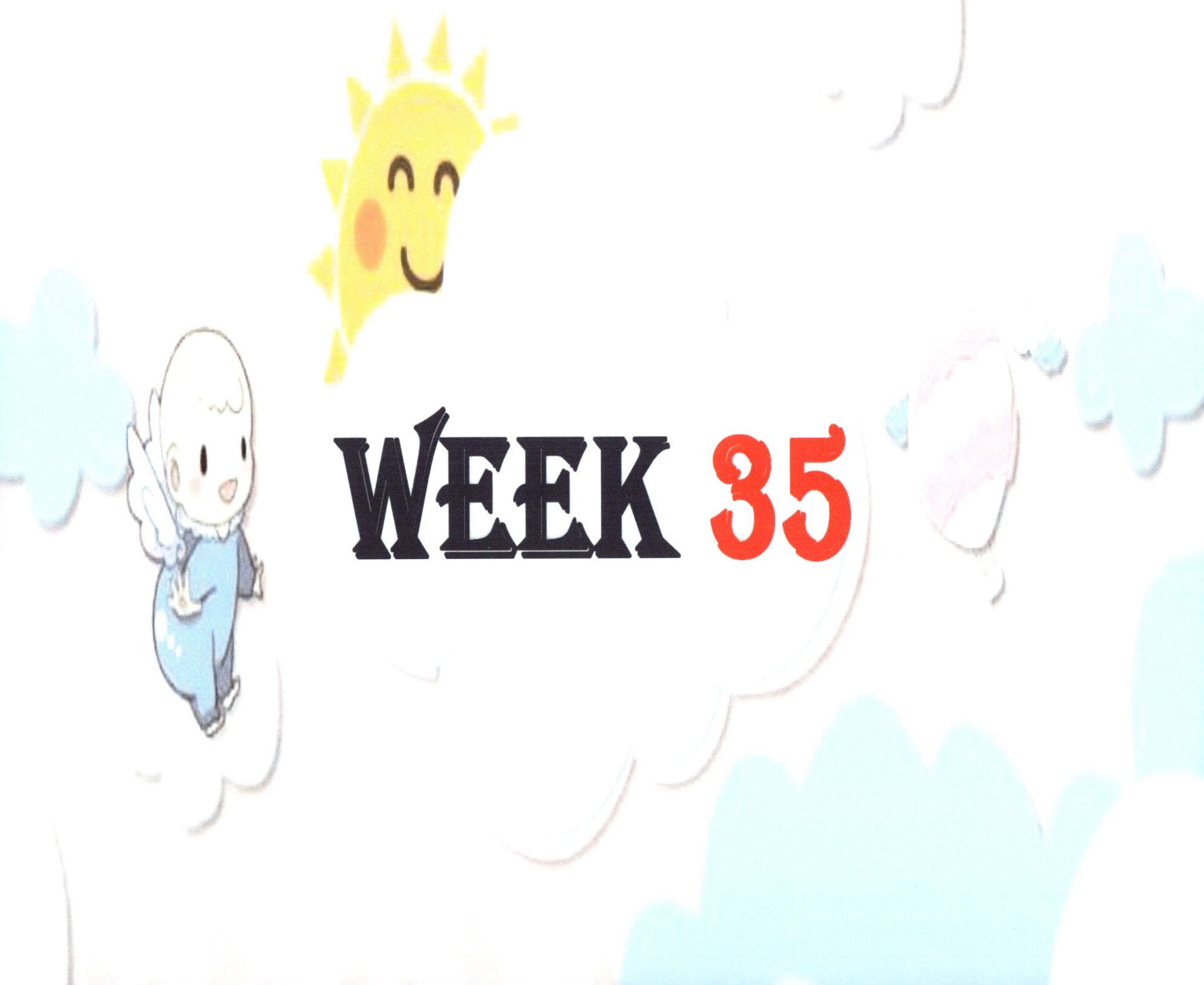

Acidity

- Acidity is a burning sensation in the chest or throat. This is due to hormonal changes in pregnancy which relax the valve between the stomach & the food pipe. Try to avoid spicy & fried foods, chocolate 7 citrus fruits like oranges, lemon & mosambi. Eat frequent small meals than a few large ones.

Catch warning signs of high blood pressure

- During this time some women may have high blood pressure or pre-eclampsia. It is important to catch the warning signs of this condition at the right time & report to your gynecologist immediately.

- Problems like headache, eyesight problems or seeing spots, breathing difficulty or pain in the shoulders or abdomen should be reported to your doctor.

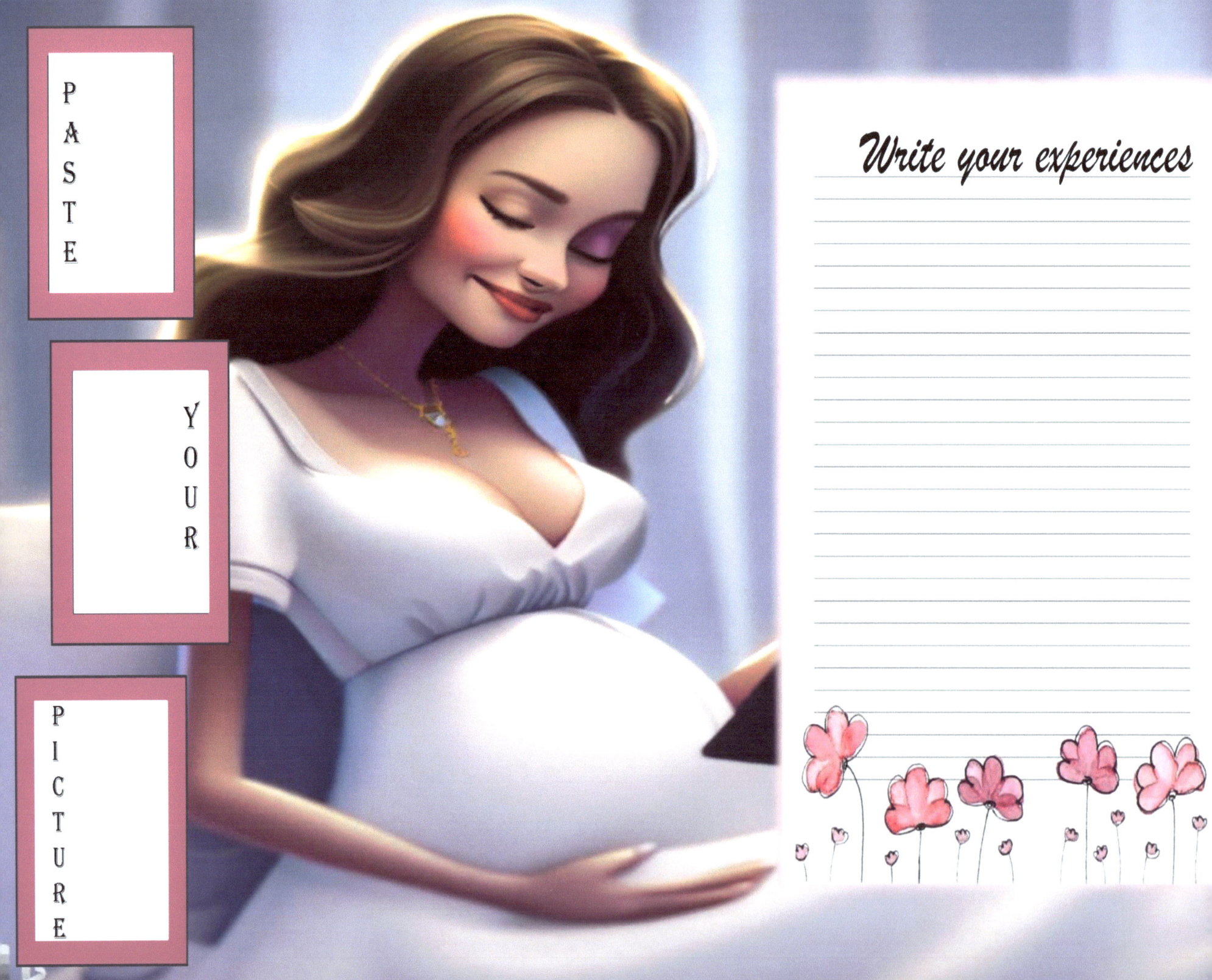

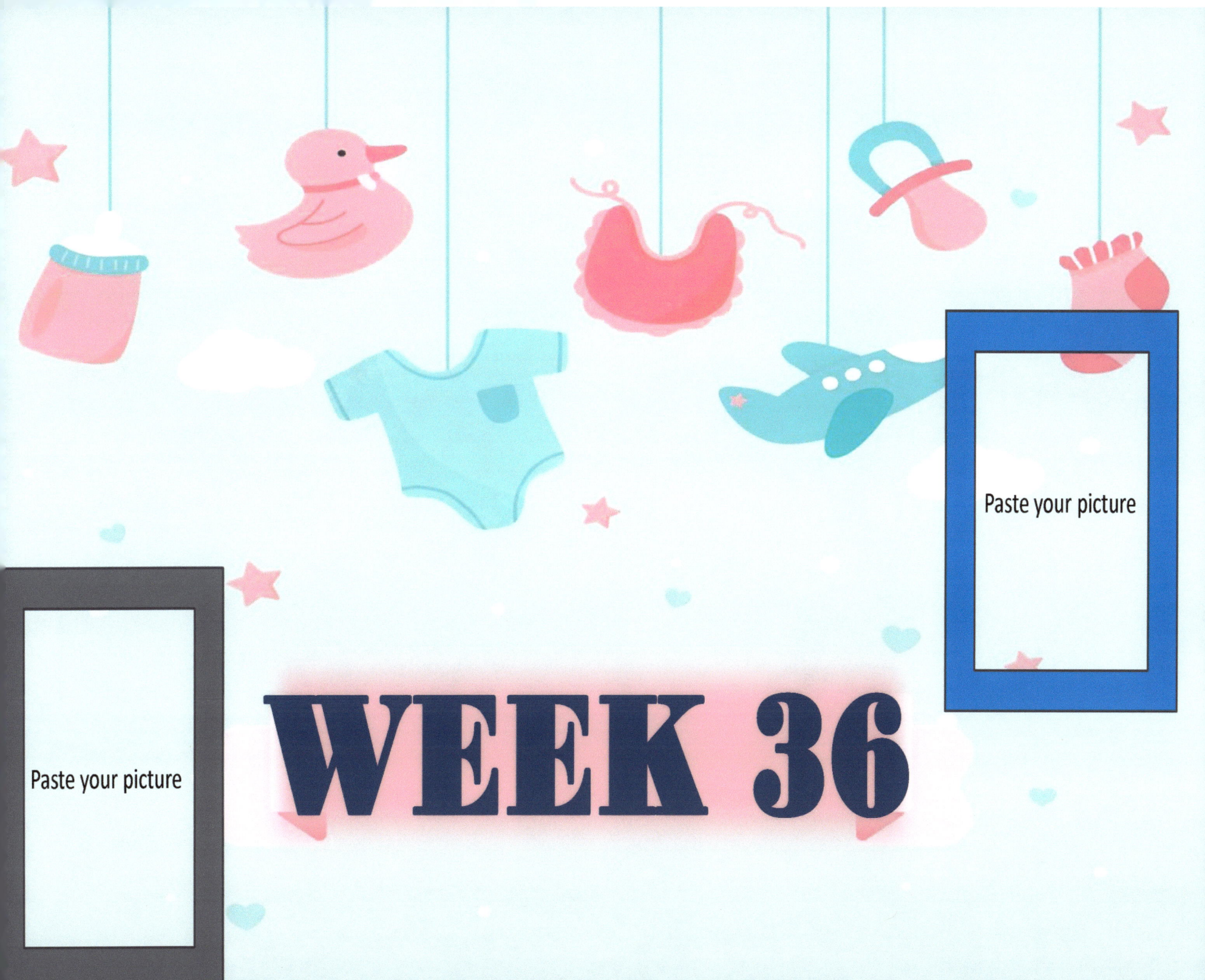

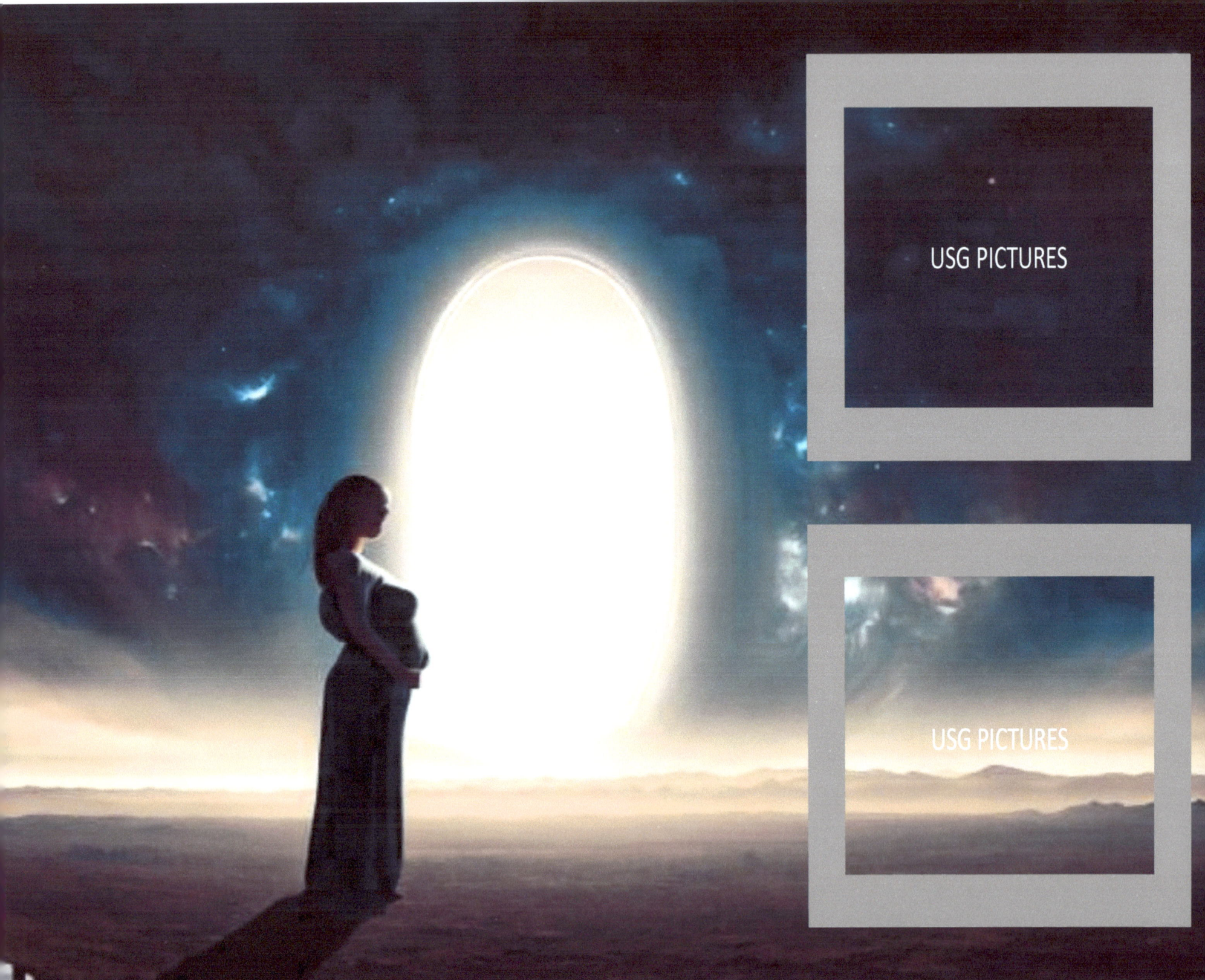

ARE YOU ACTIVE IN LABOUR?

- Active labour is the time when you notice strong signs. Shortly before delivery, the amniotic sac is broken & fluids are released. This is called water breaking. contact your doctor immediately when the happens.

- Apart from this, you feel strong uterine contractions over the lower abdominal area. These contractions increase in number, frequency, & intensity. You may feel cramps in your legs, back pain & feeling of vomiting.

DIFFERENCE BETWEEN TRUE & FALSE LABOUR

🙂 In true labour, Intervals of one contraction in every 8 to 10 mins, false labour has an irregular pattern. False labour does not get stronger or high in frequency over time.

🙂 Change in position or activity cause slowing or stopping of false labour contractions, while true labour contractions persist.

Eat plenty of greens & Drink lots of water

- Your diet is the best way of nourishing your baby while they are in the womb.

- Make sure you are eating lots of fruit and vegetables as part of a balanced diet.

- Staying hydrated is really important for both of you. Try taking a water bottle with you whenever you go.

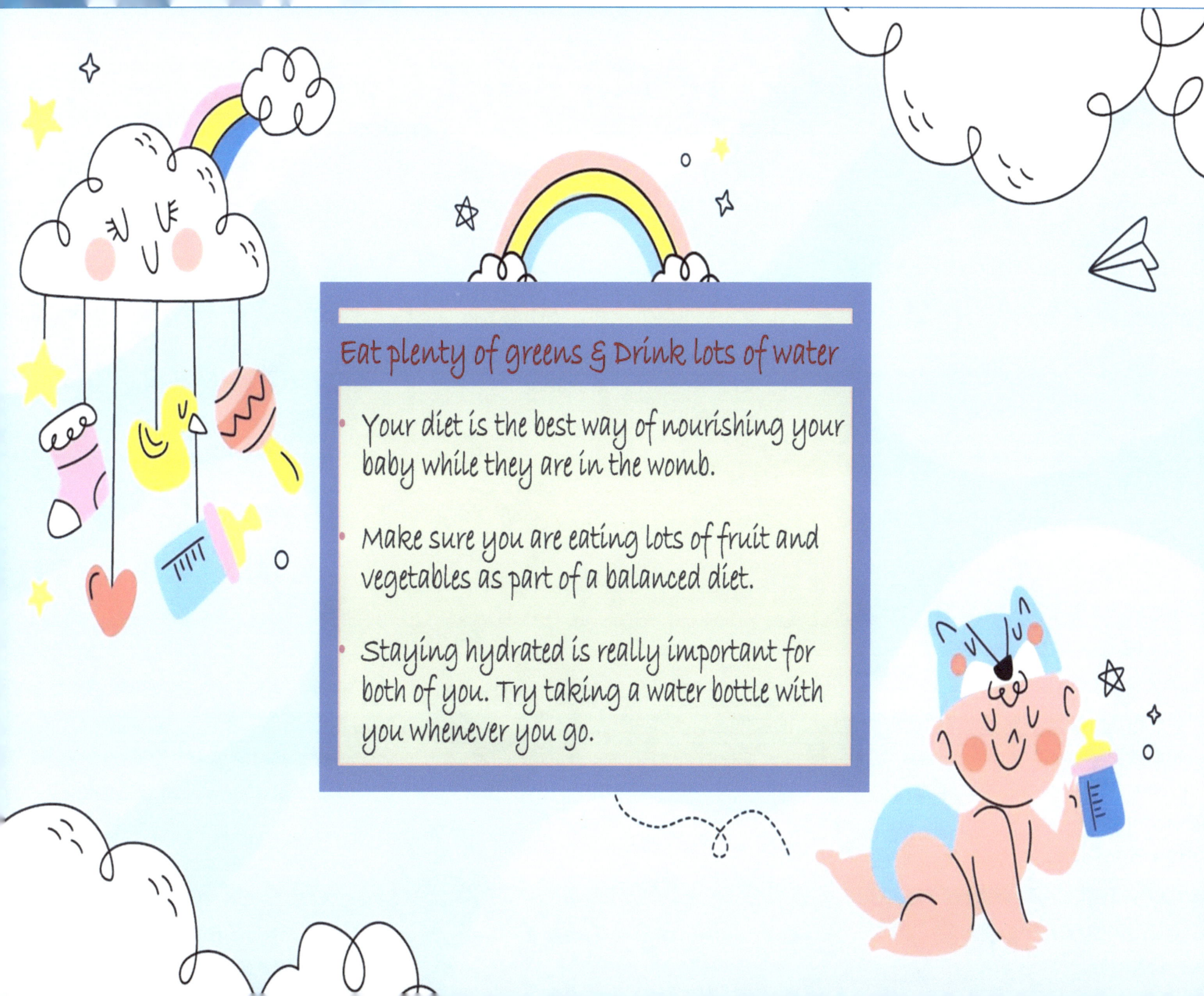

STAGES OF NORMAL LABOUR

INTRODUCTION
- Labour refers to the process of childbirth, involving the progressive opening of the cervix and the delivery of the baby.
- Labour is typically divided into four stages, each characterized by different physical and emotional changes.

STAGE 1: EARLY LABOUR
- This stage is characterized by the onset of regular contractions, which gradually become stronger and closer together.
- The cervix begins to dilate and efface (thin out).
- Women may experience backache, mild cramping, and a bloody show.
- This stage can last for several hours or even days.

STAGE 1: ACTIVE LABOUR
- Active labour begins when the cervix is around 6 centimeters dilated.
- Contractions become more intense and frequent, typically lasting 40-60 seconds and occurring every 3-5 minutes.
- Women may feel increased pressure and a strong urge to push.
- This stage usually lasts between 3 to 7 hours for first-time mothers and can be shorter for women who have given birth before.

STAGE 2: DELIVERY OF THE BABY
- This stage begins when the cervix is fully dilated (10 centimeters).
- Women may feel a strong urge to push as the baby's head descends through the birth canal.
- The baby's head crowns as it emerges, followed by the rest of the body.
- This stage typically lasts from a few minutes to a couple of hours.

STAGE 3: DELIVERY OF THE PLACENTA
- After the baby is born, the uterus continues to contract, causing the placenta to detach from the uterine wall.
- The placenta is delivered through the birth canal, usually within 15-30 minutes after the baby's birth.
- Healthcare providers may assist by gently pulling on the umbilical cord.
- This stage is relatively short and is often accompanied by a sense of relief.

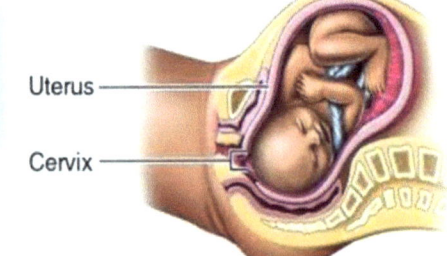

Stage 1: The cervix relaxes, causing it to dilate and thin out.

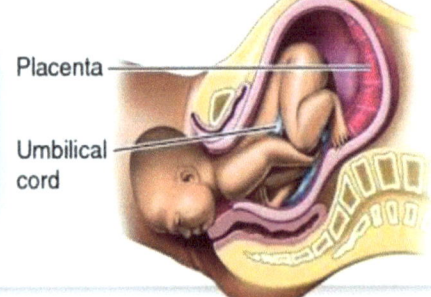

Stage 2: Uterine contractions increase in strength and the infant is delivered.

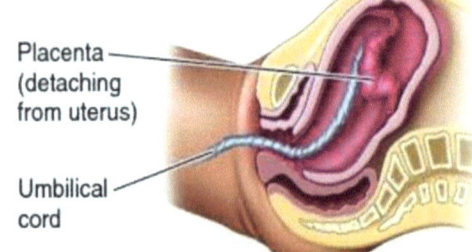

Stage 3: The placenta is expelled.

STAGES OF NORMAL LABOUR

STAGE 4: STAGE OF OBSERVATION
After the baby is born and placenta and membranes are delivered it is mandatory to observe the mother and the baby to ensure their wellness

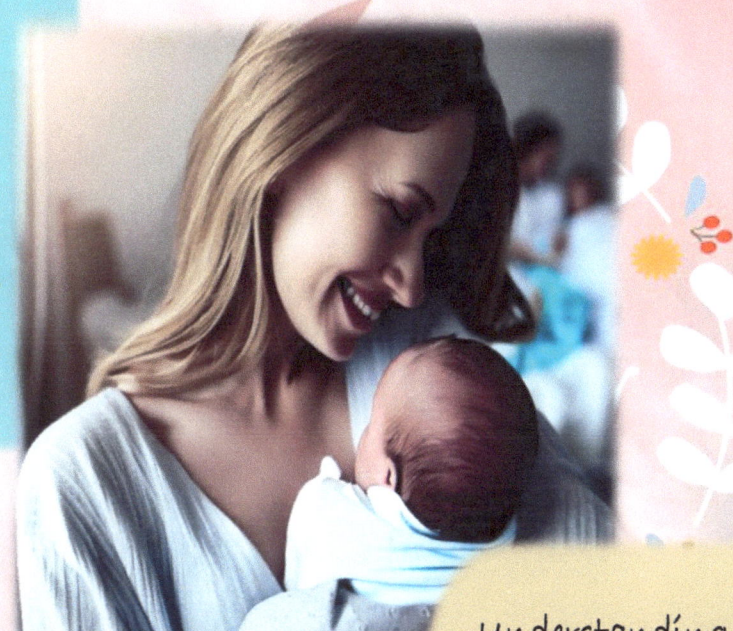

CONCLUSION
- Understanding the stages of normal labour can help expectant parents prepare for the birthing process.
- It is important to remember that every labour experience is unique, and the duration and progress of each stage can vary.
- Healthcare providers play a crucial role in supporting women during labour and ensuring a safe and positive birth experience.

BIRTH PREPAREDNESS
ENSURING A SAFE AND INFORMED BIRTH EXPERIENCE

Introduction:

Antenatal birth preparedness is a vital aspect of prenatal care that focuses on equipping expectant parents with the necessary knowledge and resources to navigate the childbirth process confidently. By understanding the importance of antenatal birth preparedness and creating a birth plan, parents can actively participate in decision-making, reduce anxiety, and enhance their overall birthing experience.

Importance of Antenatal Birth Preparedness:

1. Empowerment and Informed Decision-Making:

Antenatal birth preparedness empowers parents by providing them with comprehensive information about various aspects of childbirth. This knowledge enables expectant parents to make informed decisions regarding their birth preferences, pain management options, medical interventions, and postpartum care.

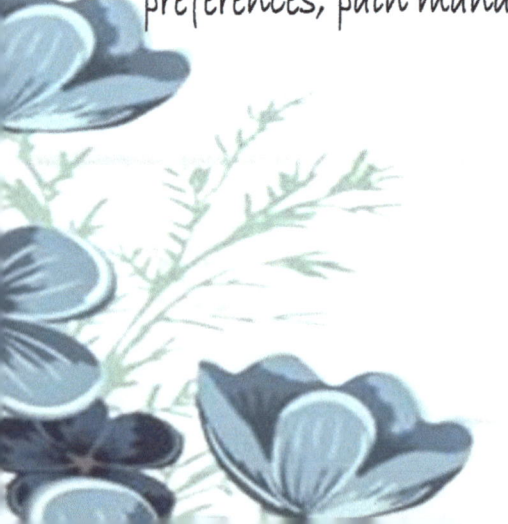
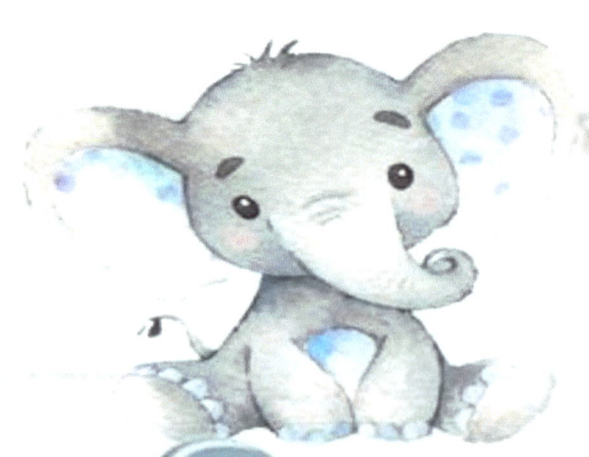
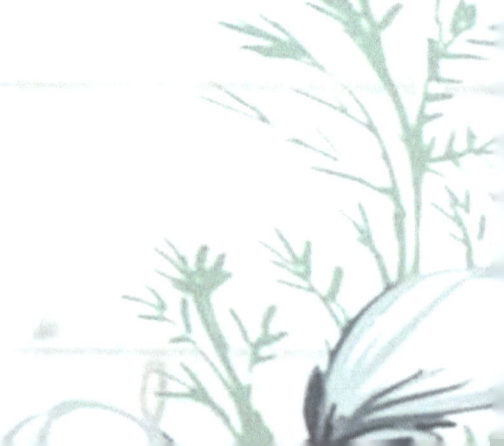

2. Reduced Anxiety and Fear:

Through antenatal education and preparation, parents can alleviate anxiety and fear surrounding childbirth. Understanding the birthing process, potential complications, and available support systems can significantly reduce stress levels and contribute to a more positive birth experience.

3. Enhanced Communication with Healthcare Providers:

Birth preparedness encourages open and effective communication between expectant parents and healthcare providers. By discussing their birth preferences, concerns, and any medical conditions, parents can establish a trusting relationship with their healthcare team, ensuring personalized care and a more supportive birth environment.

4. Preparation for Emergency Situations:

Antenatal birth preparedness also includes education on recognizing warning signs and emergency situations during childbirth. Knowing when to seek medical assistance and understanding emergency protocols can help parents respond promptly and effectively in critical situations, potentially saving lives and minimizing complications.

CREATING A BIRTH PLAN: A PROFORMA

A birth plan is a written document that outlines an expectant parent's preferences and wishes for labor, delivery, and postpartum care. While it is important to remain flexible as labor can be unpredictable, a birth plan serves as a helpful communication tool for healthcare providers. Here is a proforma to create a birth plan:

1. Personal Information:
- Name, contact details, and due date.
- Preferred language of communication.

2. Labour and Birth Preferences:
- Desired birth location (hospital, birth center, home birth).
- Preferences for pain management options (natural techniques, epidural, etc.).
- Preferred labor positions and movement during labor.
- Desire for the presence of a support person (partner, doula, family member).

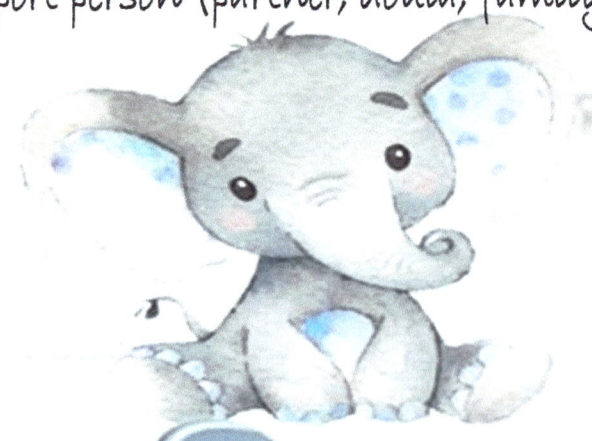

3. Monitoring and Interventions:
- Preferences for fetal monitoring methods (intermittent, continuous).
- Acceptance or refusal of specific medical interventions (induction, episiotomy, etc.).
- Preferences for assisted delivery (forceps, vacuum extraction, etc.).

4. Cesarean Birth Preferences:
- Preferences for partner presence during a cesarean section.
- Desire for immediate skin-to-skin contact with the baby after surgery.

5. Postpartum Care:
- Preferences for breastfeeding or formula feeding.
- Rooming-in with the baby or nursery care.
- Desire for early discharge or extended hospital stay.

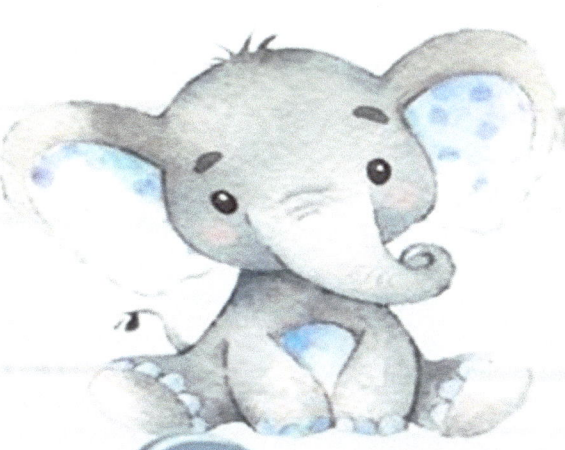
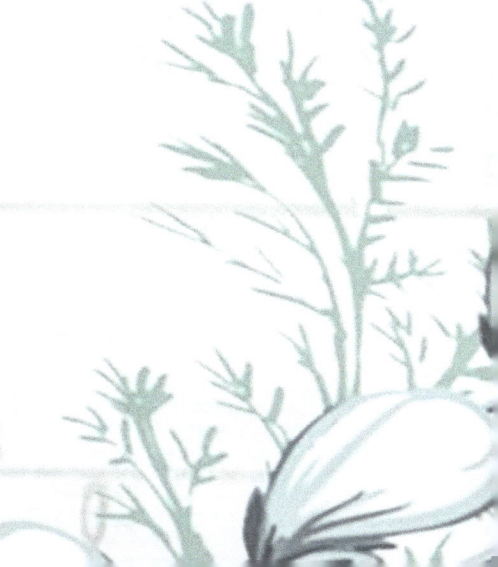

6. Special Requests or Cultural Considerations:
- Any specific cultural or religious preferences or rituals to be followed.
- Requests for photography or videography during labor and delivery.

Conclusion:

Antenatal birth preparedness is essential for expectant parents to navigate the childbirth process with confidence and active participation. By creating a birth plan, parents can effectively communicate their preferences, reduce anxiety, and ensure a personalized and positive birth experience. It is important to discuss the birth plan with healthcare providers to ensure alignment and flexibility during the labor and delivery process.

EXERCISE IN PREGNANCY

Weeks 37-40

As you near the end of your pregnancy, focus on gentle exercises that support relaxation and prepare for labor, such as prenatal yoga or meditation. Walking and swimming can continue to be beneficial for maintaining cardiovascular fitness. Listen to your body and reduce intensity if necessary.

Remember to always listen to your body, stay hydrated, and avoid overexertion or activities that cause discomfort. It's essential to modify exercises as your pregnancy progresses and seek guidance from a certified prenatal fitness instructor or healthcare provider for personalized advice.

WEEK 37

DID YOU FORGET YOUR DUE DATE???

The term due date or EDD (expected date of delivery) is deducted by a formula by your Gynaecologist and it cant be changed with each USG finding. Knowing when your baby has been gestating for 40 ½ weeks is great. But it does not tell anything about when your baby will arrive.
Don't count down to it.

GET LOADS OF REST

You probably don't need to be told to do this one! You are about to go through a very physically challenging experience, and you're probably feeling exhausted anyway. Put your feet & try to relax as much as u can.

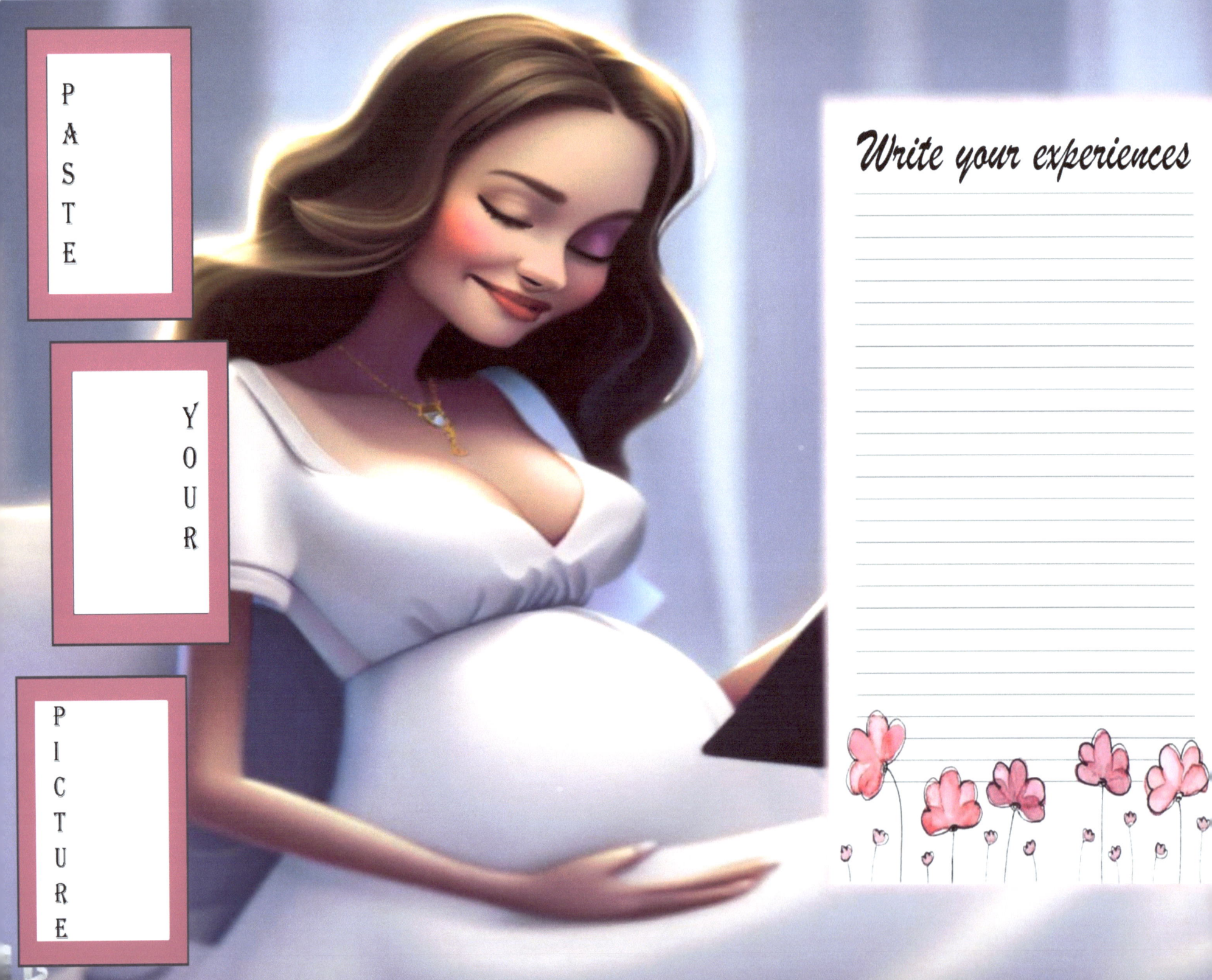

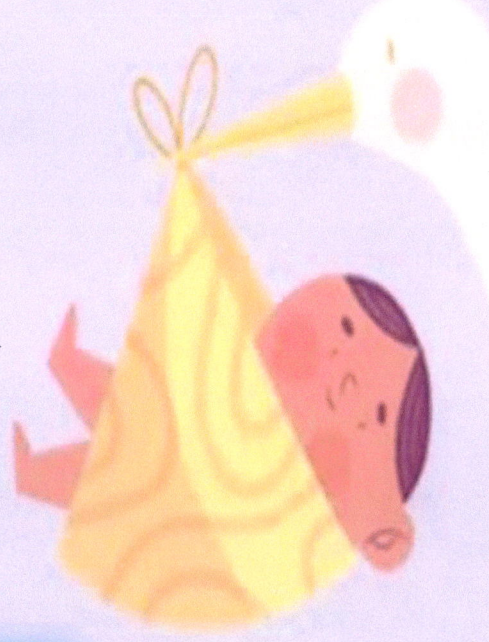

Welcome to the World!

WEEK 38

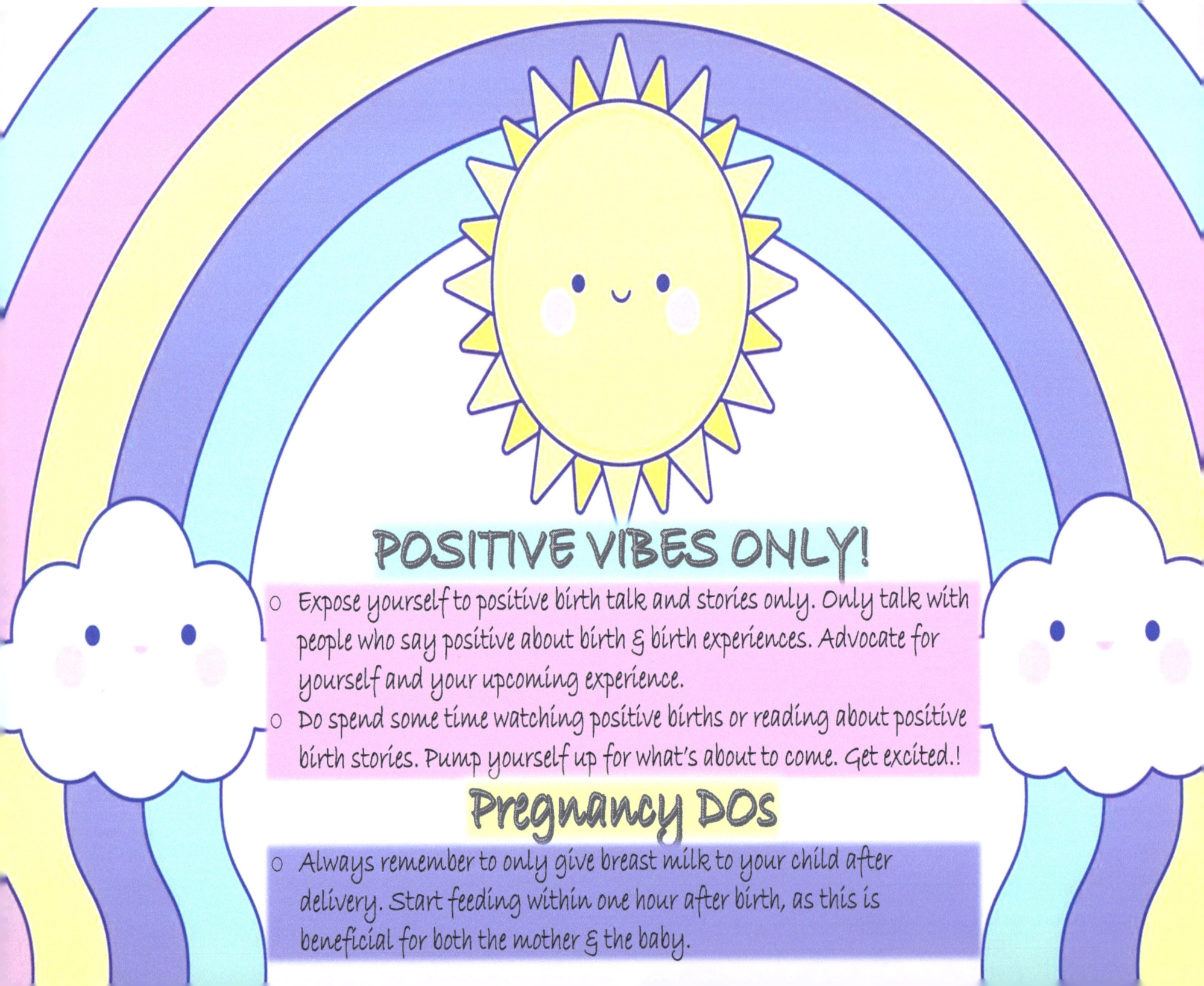

POSITIVE VIBES ONLY!

- Expose yourself to positive birth talk and stories only. Only talk with people who say positive about birth & birth experiences. Advocate for yourself and your upcoming experience.
- Do spend some time watching positive births or reading about positive birth stories. Pump yourself up for what's about to come. Get excited.!

Pregnancy DOs

- Always remember to only give breast milk to your child after delivery. Start feeding within one hour after birth, as this is beneficial for both the mother & the baby.

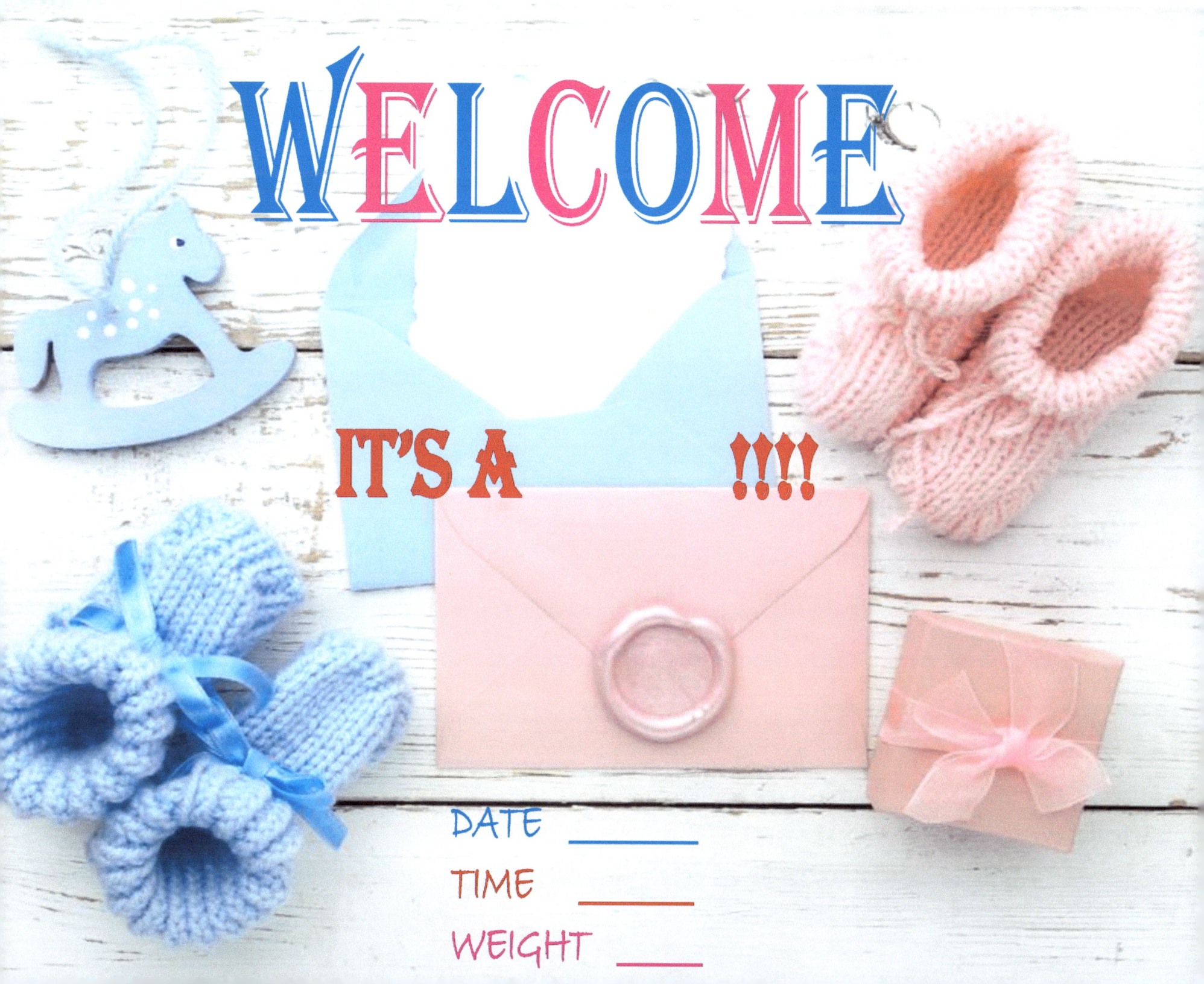

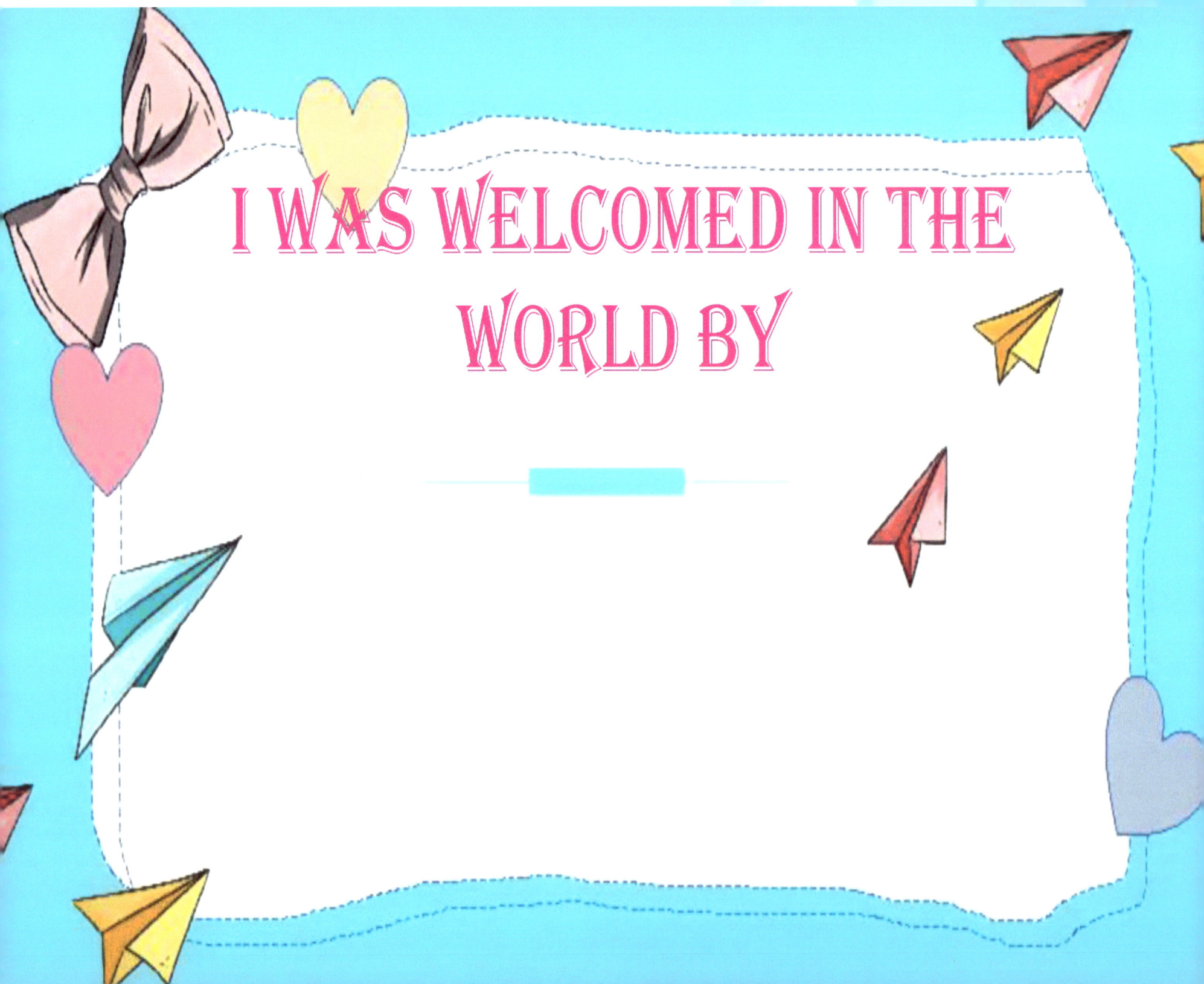

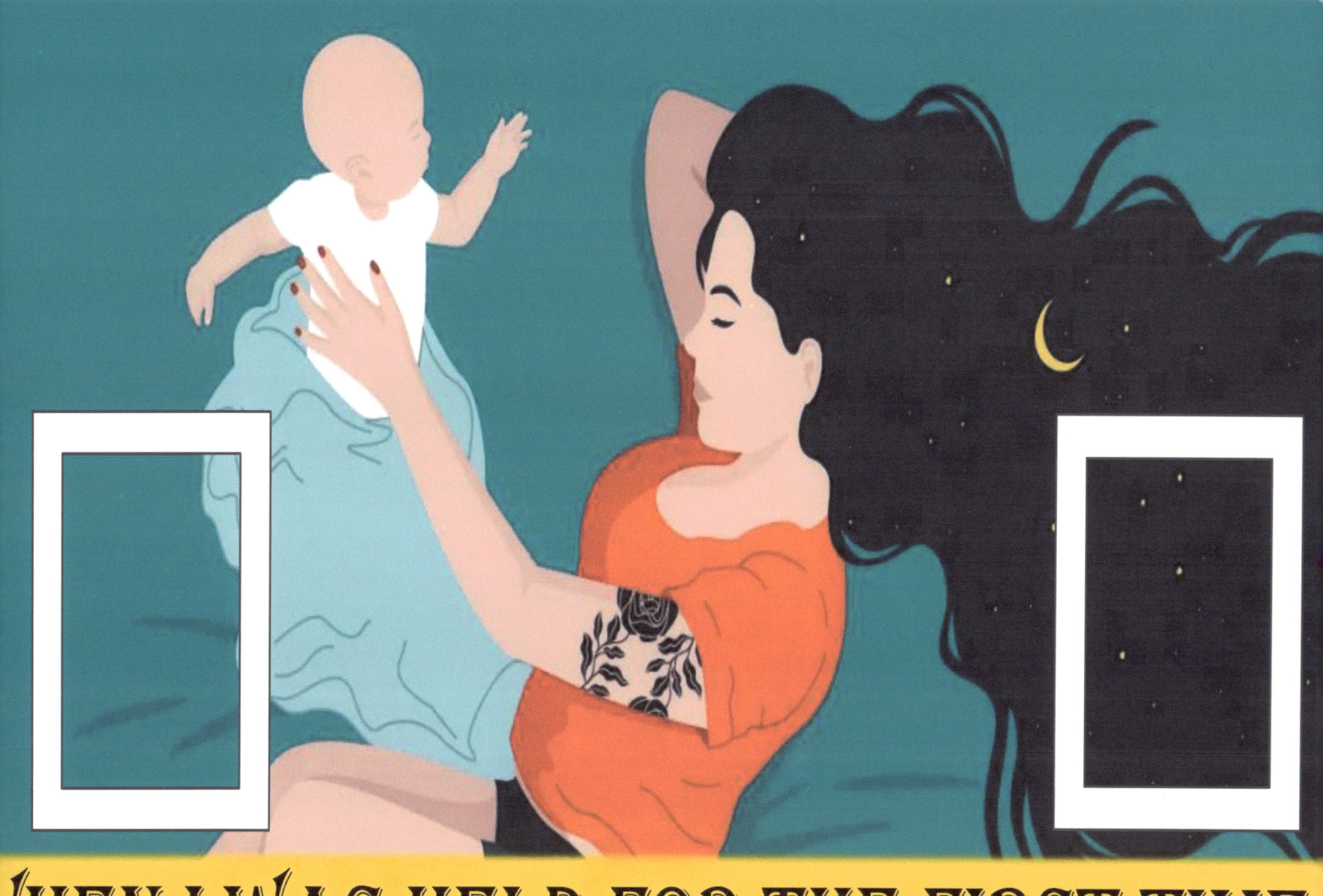

MY FIRST TOY

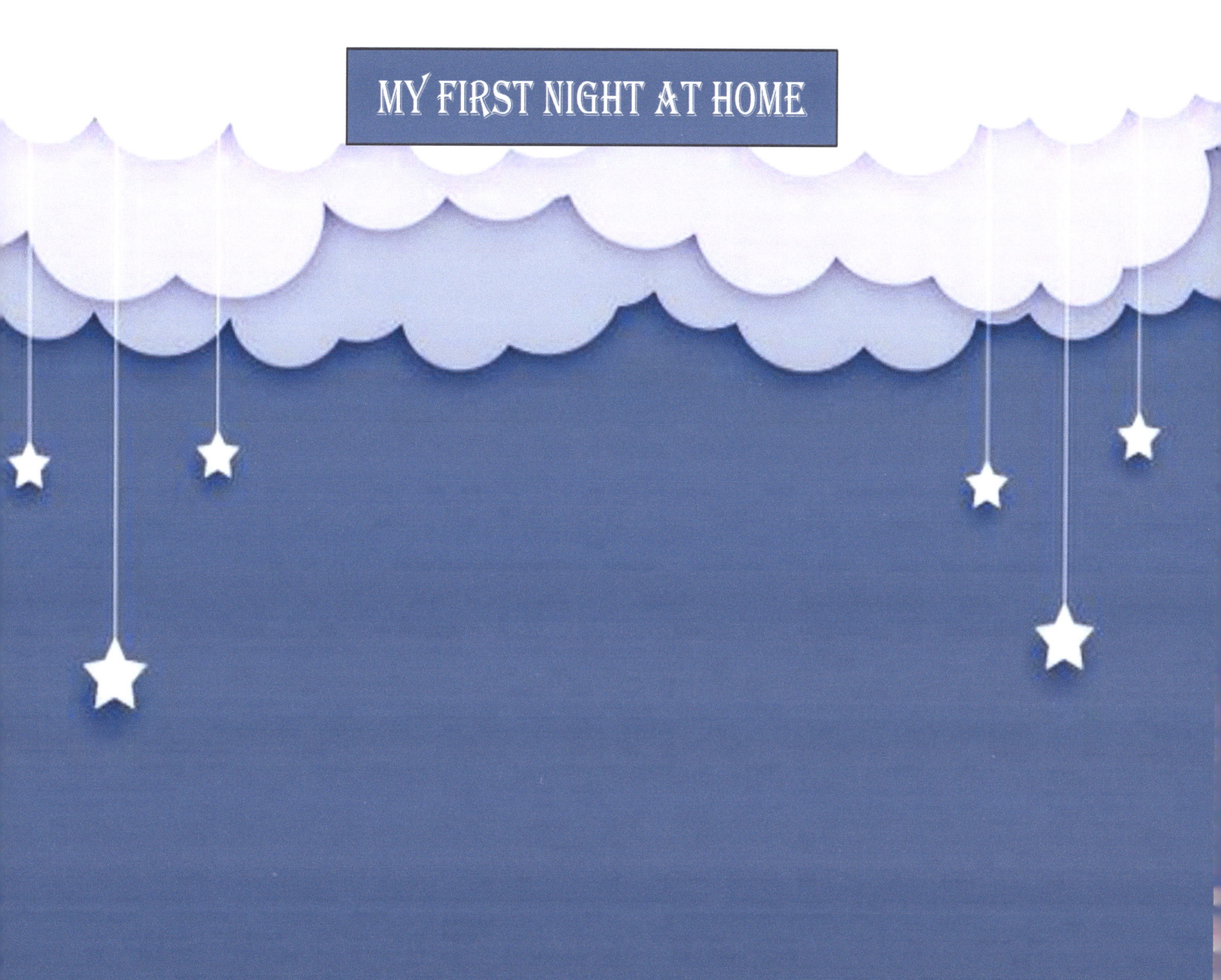

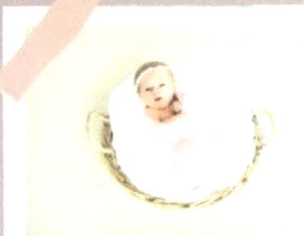 1 month
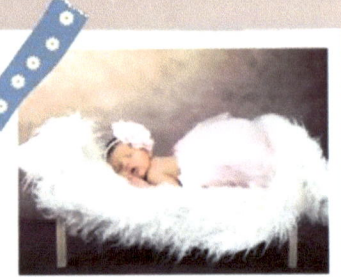 2 months
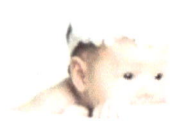 3 months
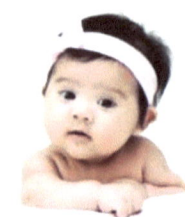 4 months
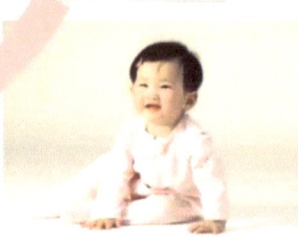 5 months
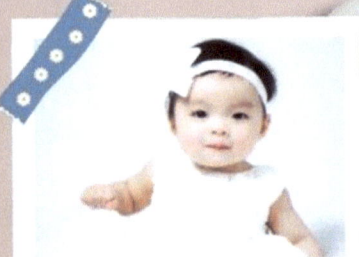 6 months
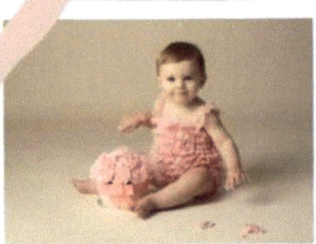 7 months
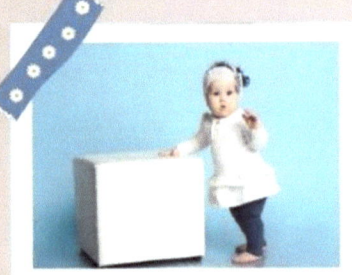 8 months
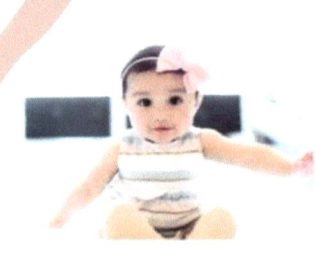 9 months
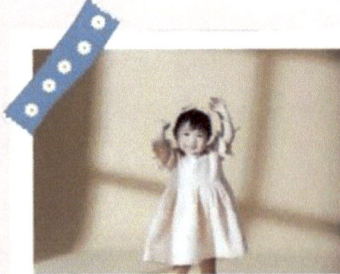 10 months
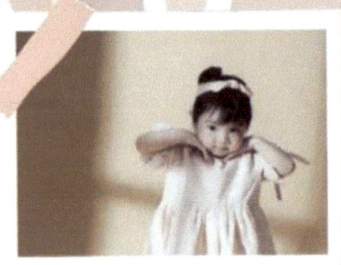 11 months
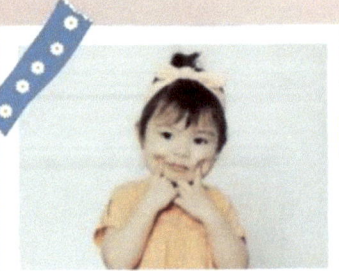 12 months

Baby

NAME

thru the months

DOS AND DON'TS AFTER NORMAL DELIVERY

DOS

- Get plenty of rest
- Practice gentle postpartum exercises
- Maintain good hygiene
- Stay hydrated
- Eat a nutritious diet
- Support your breasts while breastfeeding intervals
- Take pain medications as prescribed
- Talk to your healthcare provider about contraceptive options

DON'TS

- Don't overexert yourself
- Avoid heavy lifting or strenuous activities
- Don't ignore signs of infection, such as excessive redness or discharge
- Avoid consuming excessive caffeine or sugary drinks
- Avoid crash diets or skipping meals
- Don't ignore breastfeeding difficulties, seek help if needed
- Don't hesitate to seek medical assistance if you experience severe pain or complications
- Don't neglect your emotional well-being. Seek support if you experience postpartum blues or depression

DOS AND DON'TS AFTER CESAREAN SECTION

DOS

- Follow your healthcare provider's instructions
- Take care of your incision: Keep the incision area clean and dry to prevent infection
- Manage pain and discomfort:
- Eat a balanced diet Include foods rich in fiber, protein, vitamins, and minerals to aid in recovery
- Get enough rest, take short, frequent naps when needed and aim for quality sleep at night.

DON'TS

- Avoid lifting heavy objects during the initial weeks following a C-section, as it can strain your incision and delay healing.
- Avoid vigorous activities, intense exercises, or heavy workouts until your healthcare provider gives you the green light.
- Be vigilant for signs of infection, such as redness, swelling, warmth, discharge, or increased pain around the incision site. If you notice any concerning symptoms, notify your healthcare provider promptly.
- Neglect self-care
- Skip postpartum check-ups

BREASTFEEDING TECHNIQUES

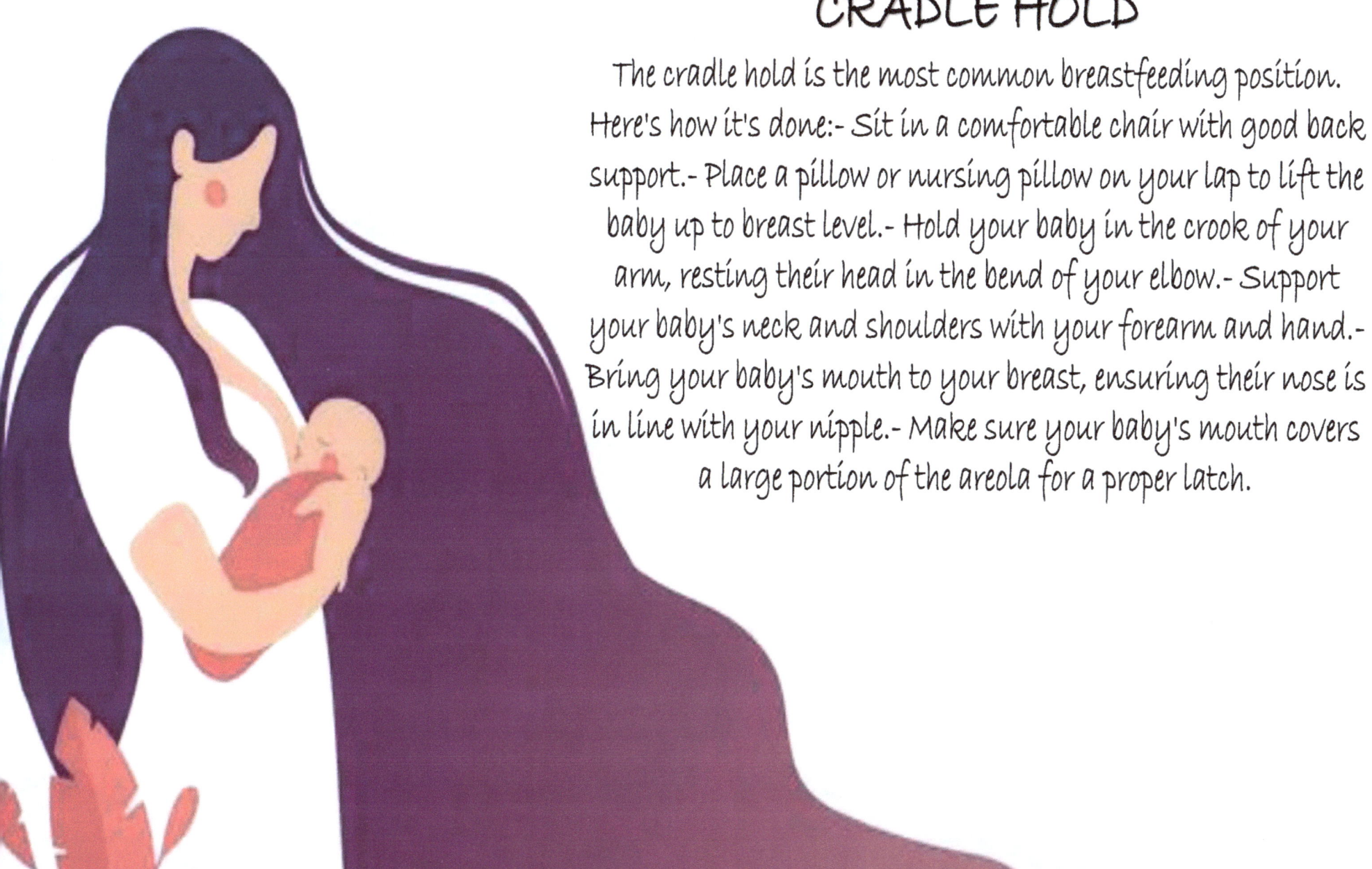

CRADLE HOLD

The cradle hold is the most common breastfeeding position. Here's how it's done:- Sit in a comfortable chair with good back support.- Place a pillow or nursing pillow on your lap to lift the baby up to breast level.- Hold your baby in the crook of your arm, resting their head in the bend of your elbow.- Support your baby's neck and shoulders with your forearm and hand.- Bring your baby's mouth to your breast, ensuring their nose is in line with your nipple.- Make sure your baby's mouth covers a large portion of the areola for a proper latch.

FOOTBALL HOLD

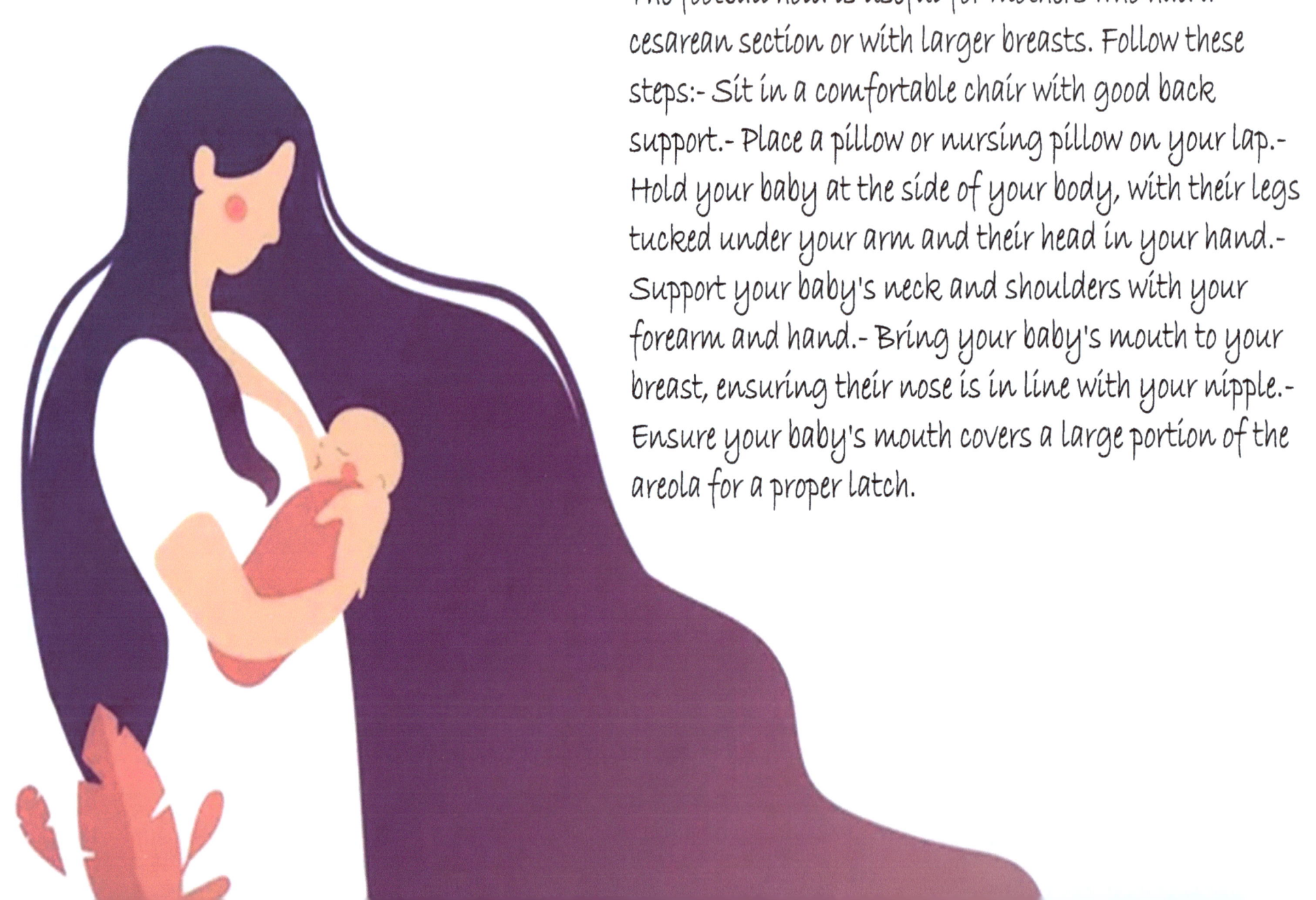

The football hold is useful for mothers who had a cesarean section or with larger breasts. Follow these steps:- Sit in a comfortable chair with good back support.- Place a pillow or nursing pillow on your lap.- Hold your baby at the side of your body, with their legs tucked under your arm and their head in your hand.- Support your baby's neck and shoulders with your forearm and hand.- Bring your baby's mouth to your breast, ensuring their nose is in line with your nipple.- Ensure your baby's mouth covers a large portion of the areola for a proper latch.

CROSS-CRADLE HOLD

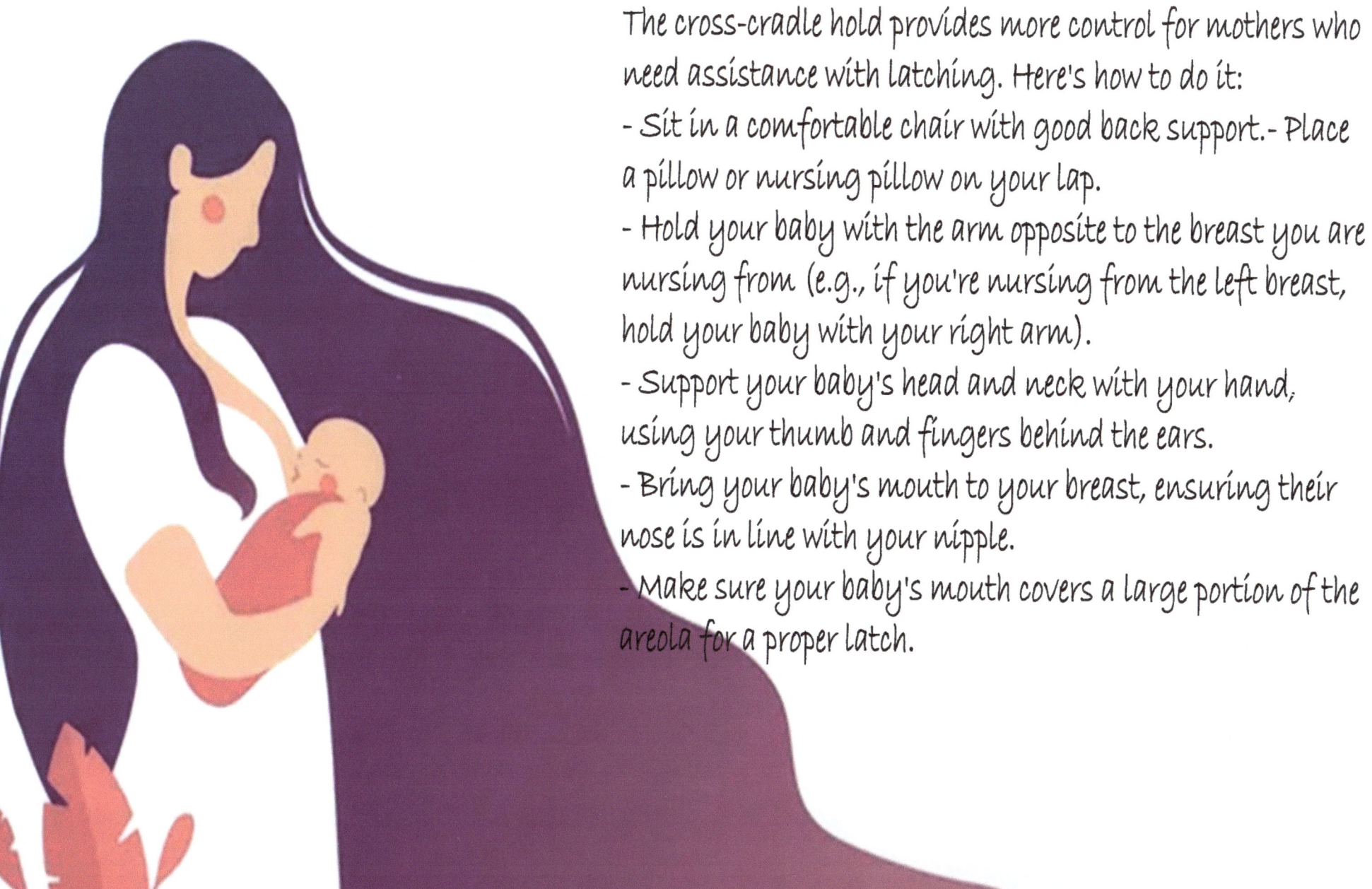

The cross-cradle hold provides more control for mothers who need assistance with latching. Here's how to do it:

- Sit in a comfortable chair with good back support.- Place a pillow or nursing pillow on your lap.
- Hold your baby with the arm opposite to the breast you are nursing from (e.g., if you're nursing from the left breast, hold your baby with your right arm).
- Support your baby's head and neck with your hand, using your thumb and fingers behind the ears.
- Bring your baby's mouth to your breast, ensuring their nose is in line with your nipple.
- Make sure your baby's mouth covers a large portion of the areola for a proper latch.

SIDE-LYING POSITION

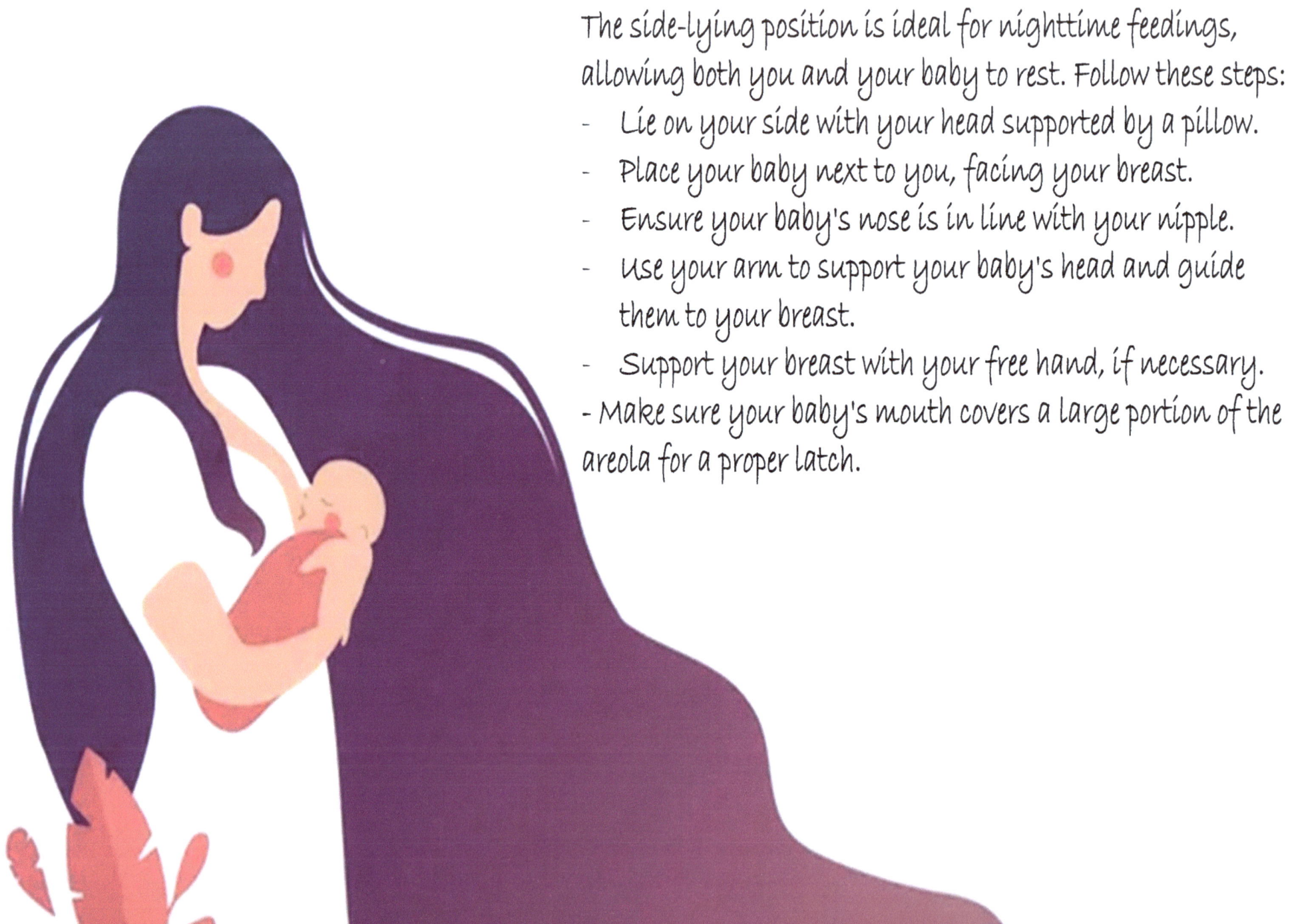

The side-lying position is ideal for nighttime feedings, allowing both you and your baby to rest. Follow these steps:
- Lie on your side with your head supported by a pillow.
- Place your baby next to you, facing your breast.
- Ensure your baby's nose is in line with your nipple.
- Use your arm to support your baby's head and guide them to your breast.
- Support your breast with your free hand, if necessary.
- Make sure your baby's mouth covers a large portion of the areola for a proper latch.

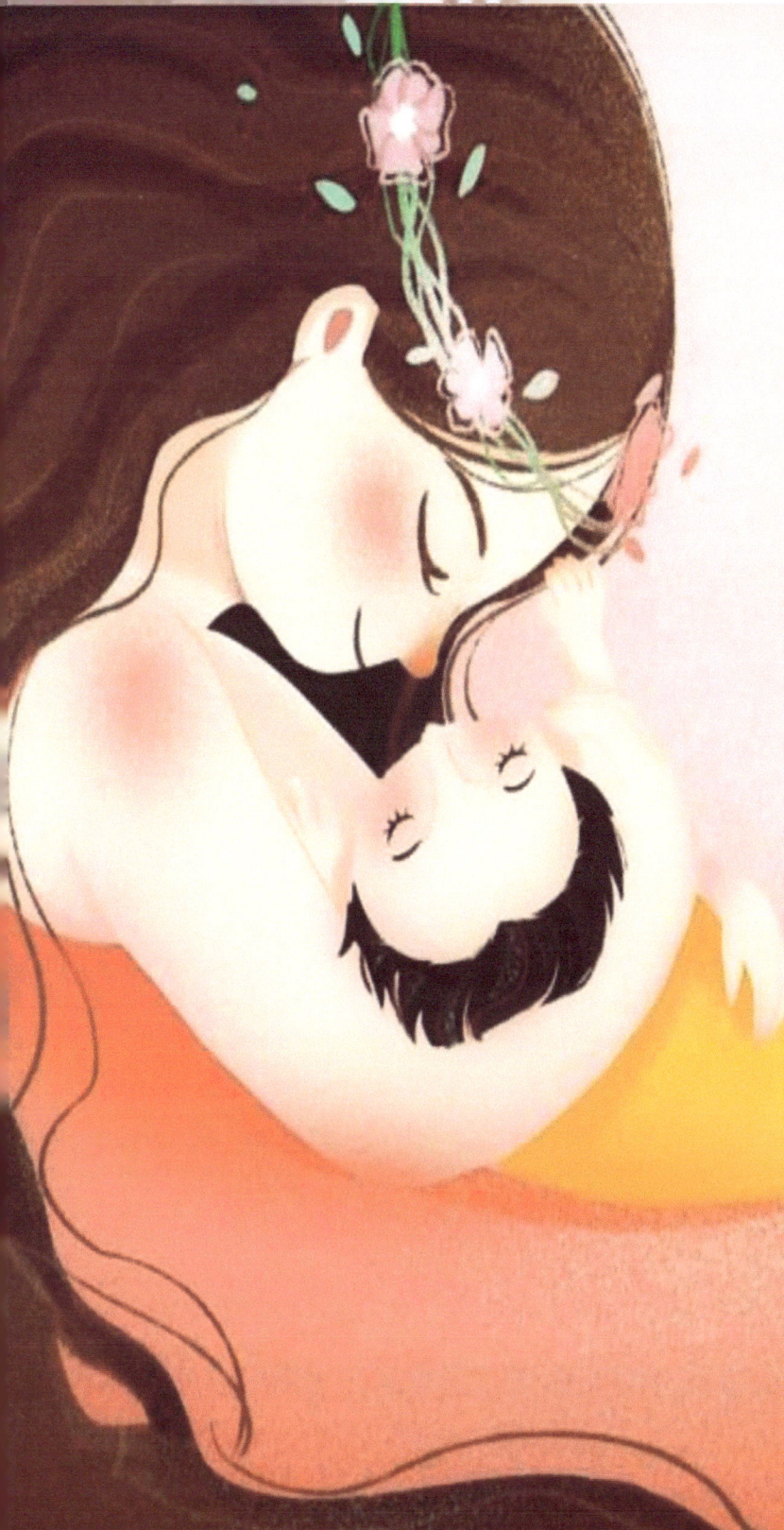

POST PARTUM CARE

Post partum is very important as it states your process of recovery from labour & delivery.

It gives a window of opportunity to the caregiver for hollistic improvement of physical, social, emotional health.

Only 58% of women go to their postnatal visits and only 28% bring babies for a postnatal check-up.

The world health organization suggests that you and your new born should have at least 3 post partum visits after delivery.

- 1st visit (could be a home visit) - within 1 week, preferably on day 3
- 2nd visit - 7 to 14 days after birth.
- 3rd visit - 4-6 weeks after birth.

It will include

- Checking in on your recovery process. (healthy stitches, involution of uterus)
- Discussion of normal post partum bleeding and lochia.

- Every woman bleeds as they give birth
- This is known as lochia
- Which is as mixture of mucous, tissue and blood that uterus sheds as it repair it's lining after childbirth.
- It often last for 4 to 6 weeks but could be upto 12 weeks.

Day1 - fresh red to brownish red, one or two clots, heavy flow may need to change pad few hourly.

Day 2-6 - Dark brown or pinkish red, smaller blood clots 7-12 cm stain on maternity pad.

Day 7-10 - Darker brown or lighter.

Day 11-14 - Darker brown becoming lighter

Week 3-4 - Creamy white blood loss, lighter flow.

Week 5-6 - pinkish, red, Creamy, yellow

If you are having large blood clots in first 24 hours,

Talk to your doctor immediately, because it could be LIFE THREATENING.

So don't keep quiet about your clots.

THE RISK FACTORS FOR PRIMARY POST PARTUM HEMORRHAGE

1. Before labour
- Previous PPH
- BMI : >35
- Twin/ Triplets pregnancy
- Low lying placenta
- Placental abruption
- Preeclampsia
- Anemia
- Taking blood thinning medication
- Blood clotting problem
- Growth in uterus (fibroid)

2. During labour
- Cesarean section
- Induced labour
- Retained placenta
- Episiotomy
- Forceps/ vaccum assisted vaginal delivery
- Labour lasted >12 hrs.
- Baby weight >4 kg
- Elderly primi > 40 yr old
- Increased temperature during labour.

3. The importance of rest, sleep
- New mom should get at least seven hours sleep.
- Full recovery can take 6 months.
- Sleep is important to combat Post partum depression.
- Optimum position is on your back.
- Place pillow under your legs to support your lower back
- Usual activities such as walking, climbing the stairs & light household work are safe but do not lift heavy objects for 6 weeks.

4. Discussion in context of healthy and nutritious food.
- As healthy and balanced diet will help your body to heal.

In post partum period a woman may need 300kcal extra than in the non-pregnant state.

As well as protein (70gm)

Calcium and fluids.

Diet Advice for Post Natal Care

Please note that this is a general guide, and individual nutritional needs may vary. It's important to consult with a healthcare professional or a registered dietitian for personalized advice.

Meal 1 (Breakfast)

Option 1 (Vegetarian): Oatmeal topped with fresh fruits (such as berries or sliced bananas) or scrambled tofu. A glass of freshly squeezed orange juice or a piece of whole fruit

Option 2 (Non-vegetarian): Vegetable omelet (made with eggs or egg whites) with spinach, bell peppers, and tomatoes Whole grain toast with avocado or nut butter A glass of milk or dairy-free alternative

Meal 2 (Mid-Morning Snack)

Greek yogurt with granola and mixed nuts Hydrating beverage like coconut water or infused water

MEAL 3 (LUNCH)

Option 1 (Vegetarian): Quinoa or brown rice Grilled vegetables (such as broccoli, zucchini, and bell peppers) Lentil or chickpea salad with mixed greens Freshly squeezed lemonade or herbal tea

Option 2 (Non-vegetarian): Grilled chicken breast or fish (like salmon or tilapia) Steamed vegetables or a side salad Whole grain pasta or couscous Freshly squeezed lemonade or herbal tea

MEAL 4 (AFTERNOON SNACK):

Hummus with whole grain pita bread or veggie sticks Sliced fruits like apple or pear Herbal tea or infused water

MEAL 5 (DINNER):

Option 1 (Vegetarian): Baked sweet potato or quinoa Tofu or chickpea curry Steamed or roasted vegetables Herbal tea or warm milk with turmeric

Option 2 (Non-vegetarian): Grilled or baked chicken or fish (like trout or cod) Roasted sweet potatoes or quinoa Steamed or stir-fried vegetables Herbal tea or warm milk with turmeric

MEAL 6 (EVENING SNACK):

Nut butter or cheese with whole grain crackers Trail mix with dried fruits and nuts Herbal tea or a glass of milk or dairy-free alternative

Note: It's important for new mothers to stay well-hydrated throughout the day. Drink plenty of water and fluids like herbal tea, coconut water, or infused water.

Remember, this is just a sample diet chart, and individual dietary needs may vary. It's important to prioritize a well-balanced diet that includes a variety of nutrient-dense foods, adequate protein, healthy fats, and plenty of fruits and vegetables. Additionally, ensure that you get enough rest and seek guidance from your healthcare provider or a registered dietitian for personalized nutritional advice.

MENTAL HEALTH CARE

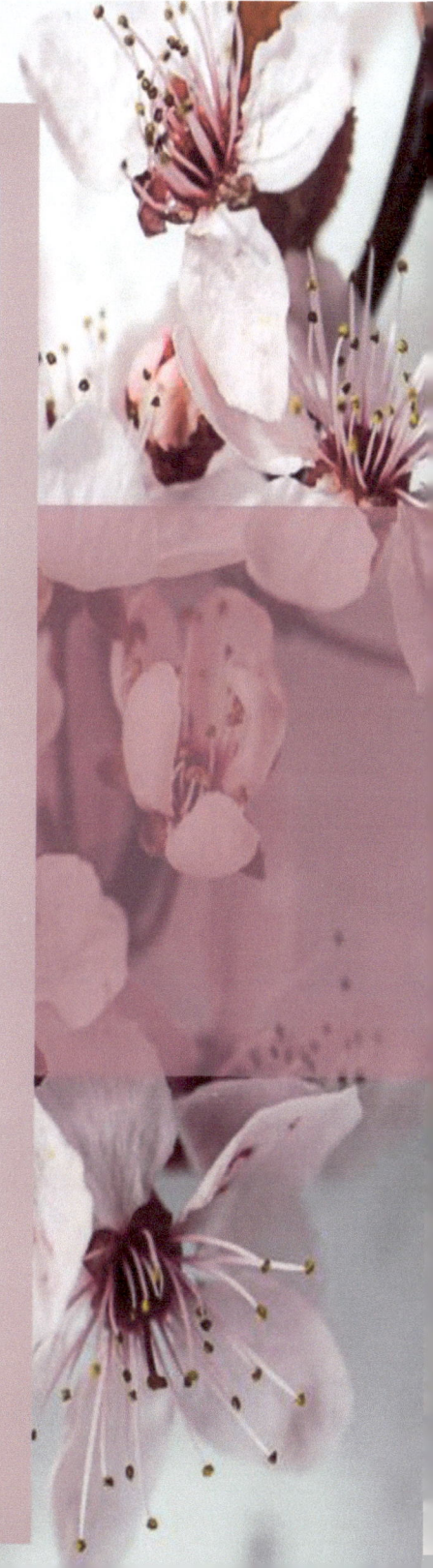

Taking care of mental health in the postpartum period is essential for new parents. Here are some ways to do so:

1. Seek support: Reach out to family, friends, or support groups who have experienced postpartum period to gain insight and find companionship.

2. Prioritize self-care: Set aside time for yourself to engage in activities that bring you joy and relaxation, like taking a walk, reading, or practicing mindfulness exercises.

3. Get enough sleep: Although challenging with a newborn, try to create a routine that allows you to get sufficient rest. Ask your partner or family members to help with nighttime feedings, if possible.

4. Maintain a healthy diet: Eating nutritious food can help improve your mood and energy levels. Avoid skipping meals, even when time is limited, and opt for foods that provide essential nutrients.

5. Exercise: Physical activity can release endorphins, which are natural mood boosters. Start with gentle exercises and gradually increase intensity over time, but always consult your healthcare provider before starting any exercise routine.

6. Accept help: Allow others to assist you with household chores, cooking, or looking after the baby, so you have some time to relax and recharge.

7. Communicate openly: Share your feelings and experiences with those close to you, including your partner, family, or friends. Honest, open communication can help alleviate stress and promote emotional well-being.

8. Join support groups: Participating in postpartum support groups or seeking professional help can provide a safe space to discuss your emotions, learn coping strategies, and receive guidance from mental health professionals.

9. Practice self-compassion: Remind yourself that it is normal to experience a range of emotions during the postpartum period. Be kind to yourself and do not judge or criticize your feelings.

10. Limit social media exposure: Social media can sometimes create unrealistic expectations or induce comparison, which can negatively affect mental health.

Take breaks from social media and focus on connecting with loved ones in person. If you notice persistent feelings of sadness, anxiety, or lack of interest in activities, it is crucial to consult your healthcare provider for further evaluation and guidance.

POSTPARTUM DEPRESSION

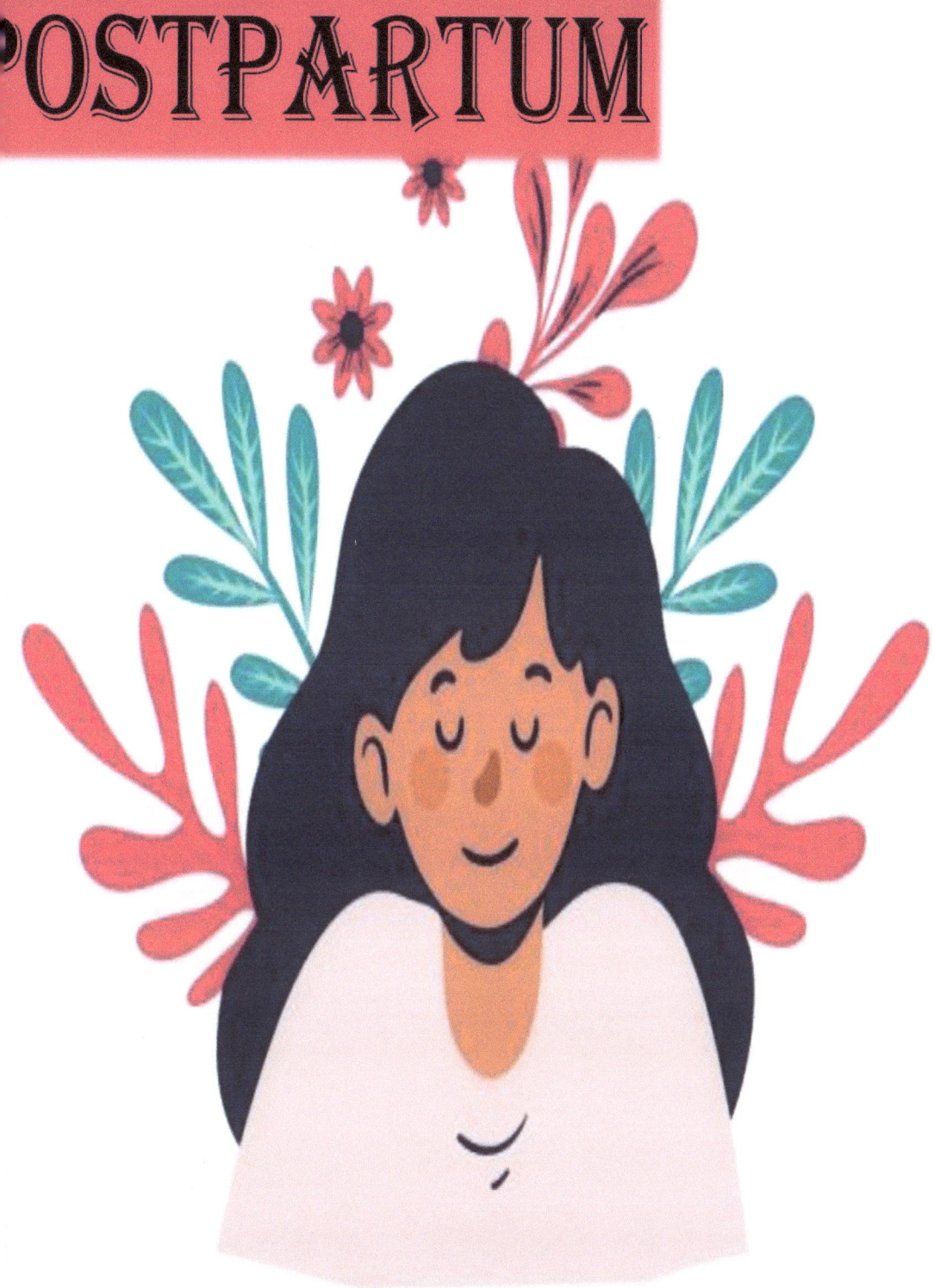

Postpartum depression and psychosis are significant mental health conditions that can affect women after childbirth. These conditions can have profound impacts on both the mother and the newborn, highlighting the importance of understanding their causes, pathogenesis, investigation, and management. In recent years, there have been numerous studies investigating these areas, providing important insights into the identification and treatment of postpartum depression and psychosis.

Causes and Pathogenesis

The causes of postpartum depression and psychosis are complex and multifactorial, involving a combination of biological, psychological, and social factors. Hormonal changes, alterations in brain chemistry, and genetic predispositions are believed to play a role in the onset of these conditions. Additionally, psychosocial factors such as a history of previous mental health issues, stressful life events, lack of social support, and difficulties adjusting to the challenges of motherhood can contribute to the development of postpartum depression and psychosis.

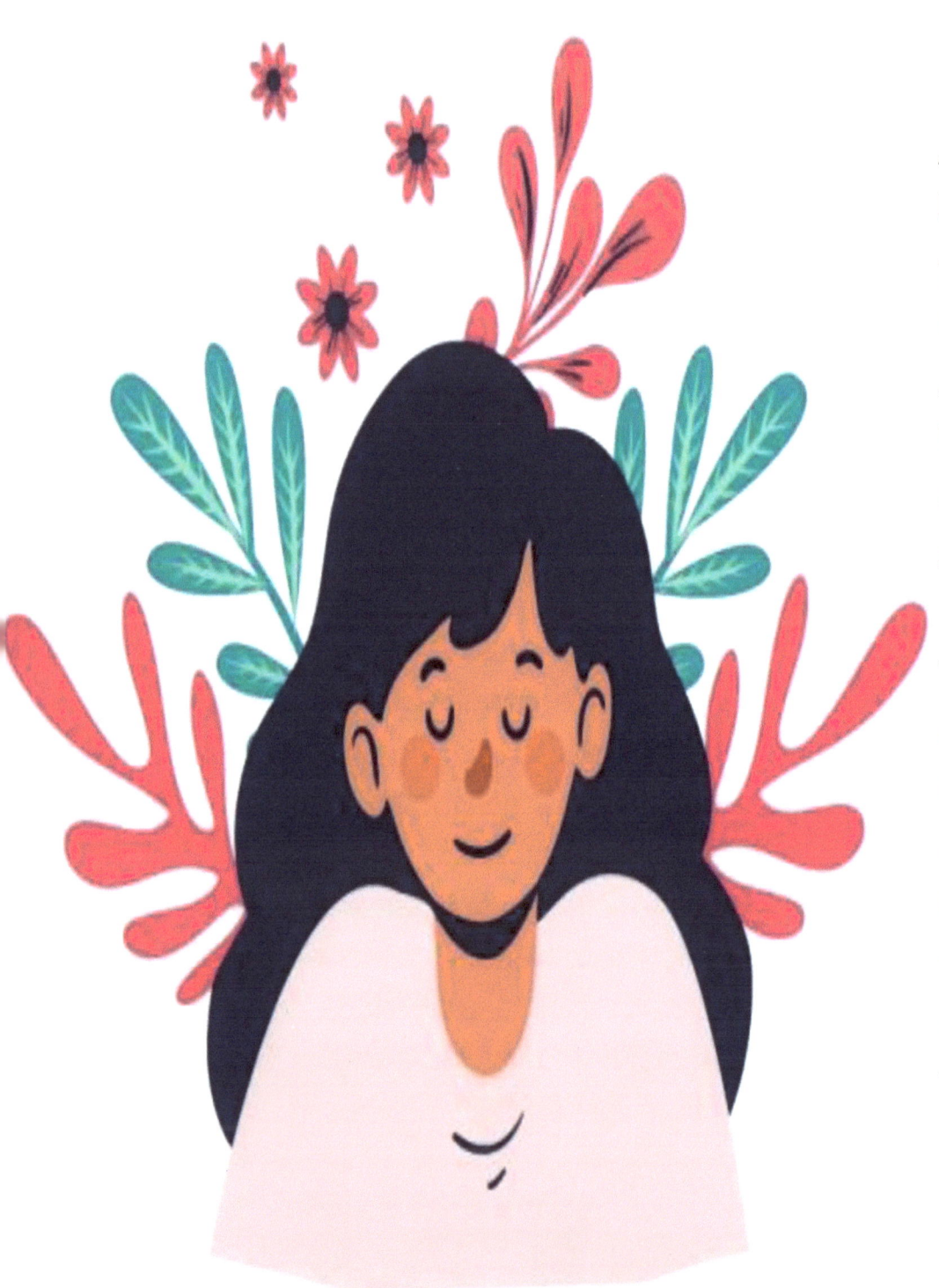

A study by Bloch et al. in 2003 investigated the role of hormones in postpartum depression and found that fluctuations in reproductive hormones during childbirth may contribute to the development of depressive symptoms. Another study by Kendell et al. in 1987 highlighted the importance of genetic factors, demonstrating a higher risk of postpartum psychosis in women with a family history severe mental illness.

Investigation

The identification and diagnosis of postpartum depression and psychosis rely on thorough clinical assessment. Healthcare professionals, particularly obstetricians, midwives, and mental health specialists, play a crucial role in recognizing and investigating these conditions. Several screening tools and scoring systems have been developed aid in the evaluation of postpartum depression and psychosis.

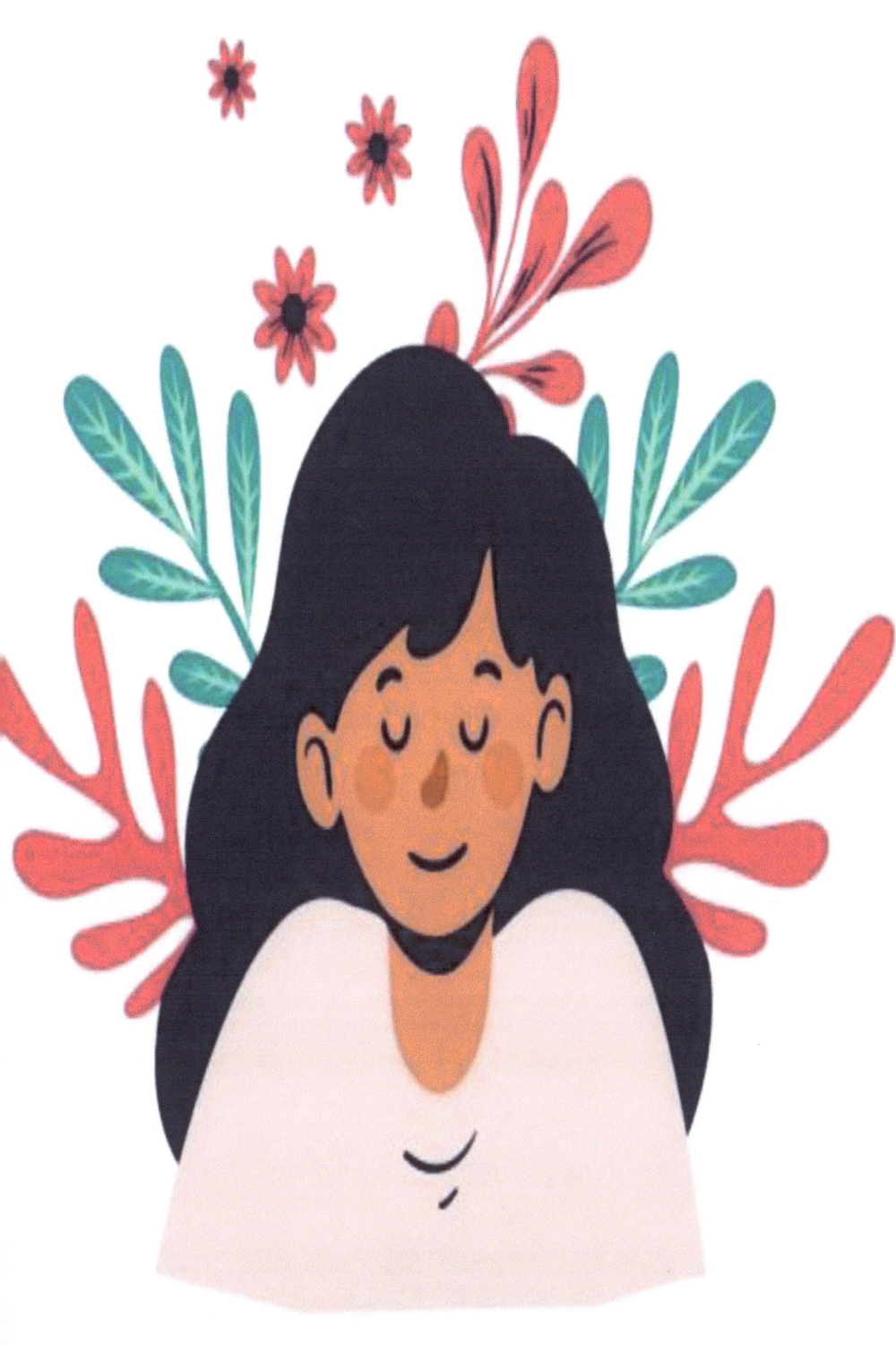

Management

The management of postpartum depression and psychosis involves a multidimensional approach that focuses on both pharmacological and non-pharmacological interventions. In mild to moderate cases, psychotherapy, support groups, and lifestyle modifications such as exercise and sleep hygiene can be beneficial. Antidepressant medications, such as selective serotonin reuptake inhibitors (SSRIs), are often prescribed in more severe cases.

In summary, postpartum depression and psychosis are complex mental health conditions that necessitate a comprehensive understanding of their causes, pathogenesis, investigation, and management. Through research and the development of scoring systems, healthcare professionals can better identify and address these conditions, ultimately improving the health and well-being of both mothers and their newborns.

CERVICAL CANCER VACCINATION AFTER DELIVERY PROTECTING YOUR HEALTH AND FUTURE

Introduction

Cervical cancer is a significant health concern that affects many women worldwide. Fortunately, advances in medical science have led to the development of effective vaccines that can prevent the most common types of cervical cancer. If you haven't received the vaccination before or during pregnancy, it's important to understand the impact and advantages of getting vaccinated after delivery. In this article, we will explore the benefits of cervical cancer vaccination, different types of vaccines available, and their possible side effects.

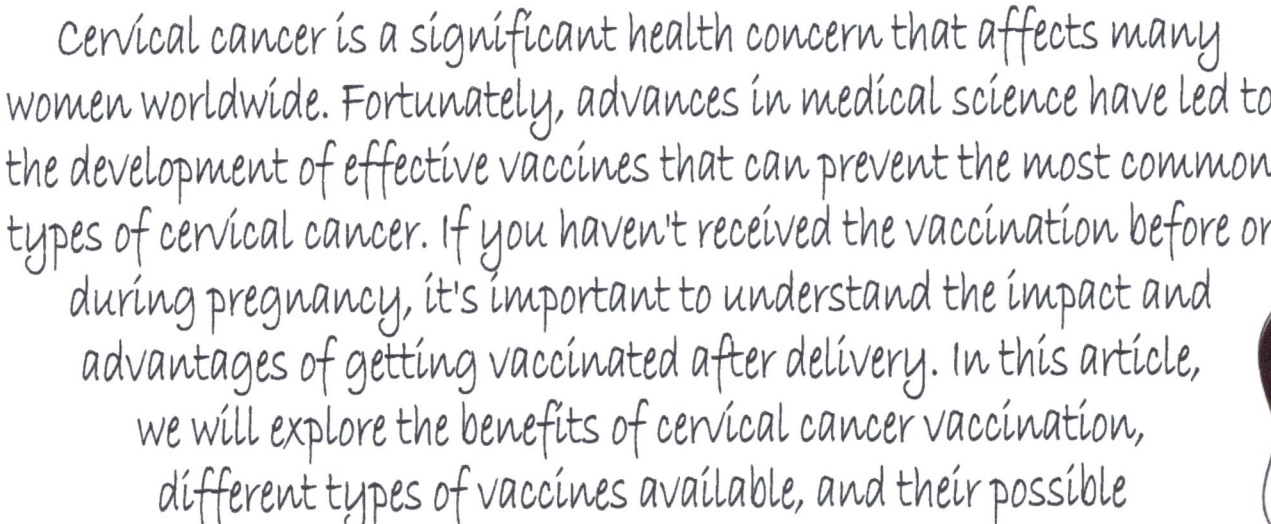

UNDERSTANDING CERVICAL CANCER AND VACCINATION

Cervical cancer is primarily caused by persistent infections with certain types of the human papillomavirus (HPV). It is one of the most preventable forms of cancer through regular screening and vaccination. HPV vaccines work by stimulating the immune system to produce antibodies that protect against HPV infection.

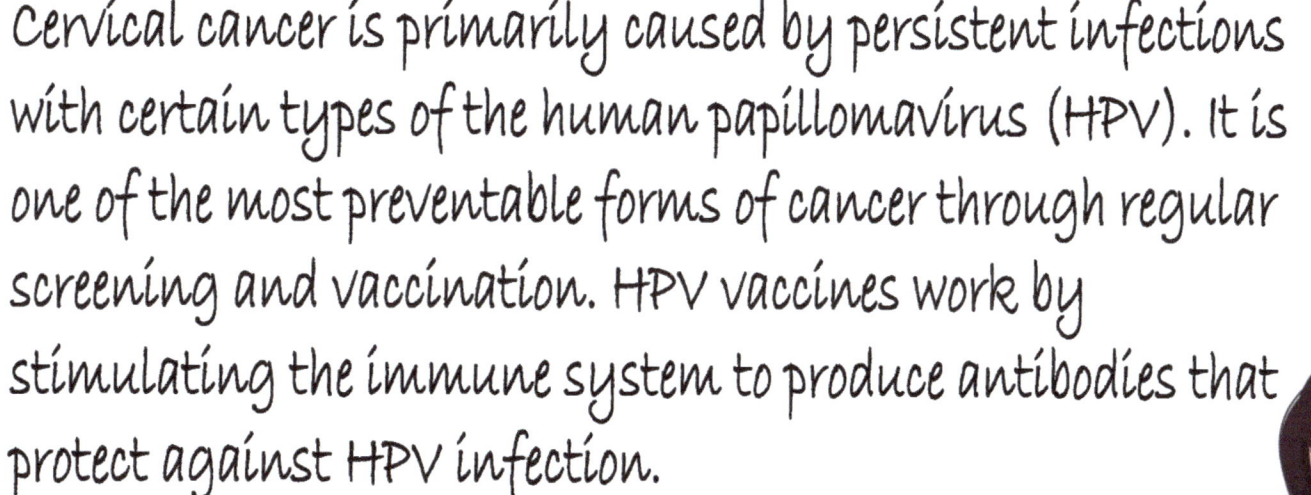

ADVANTAGES OF CERVICAL CANCER VACCINATION

Protection against HPV: The primary benefit of cervical cancer vaccination is the prevention of HPV infections, which are responsible for the majority of cervical cancer cases. By receiving the vaccine, you can reduce your risk of developing cervical cancer in the future.

Long-lasting protection: HPV vaccines provide long-term protection against the most common types of HPV that cause cervical cancer. This protection can last for many years, potentially even a lifetime, reducing the need for further interventions.

TYPES OF CERVICAL CANCER VACCINES

Gardasil: Gardasil is a widely used HPV vaccine that protects against four HPV types: 6, 11, 16, and 18. These types are responsible for causing the majority of cervical cancers, as well as other HPV-related conditions like genital warts.

Cervarix: Cervarix is another HPV vaccine that protects against HPV types 16 and 18, which are responsible for about 70% of cervical cancer cases. It does not provide protection against HPV types 6 and 11.

GETTING VACCINATED AFTER DELIVERY

If you haven't received the cervical cancer vaccination earlier, it is still recommended to get vaccinated after delivery. The vaccine can be administered during the postpartum period, even if you are breastfeeding. By getting vaccinated, you not only protect yourself from future HPV infections and cervical cancer but also create a safer environment for your baby's health and well-being.

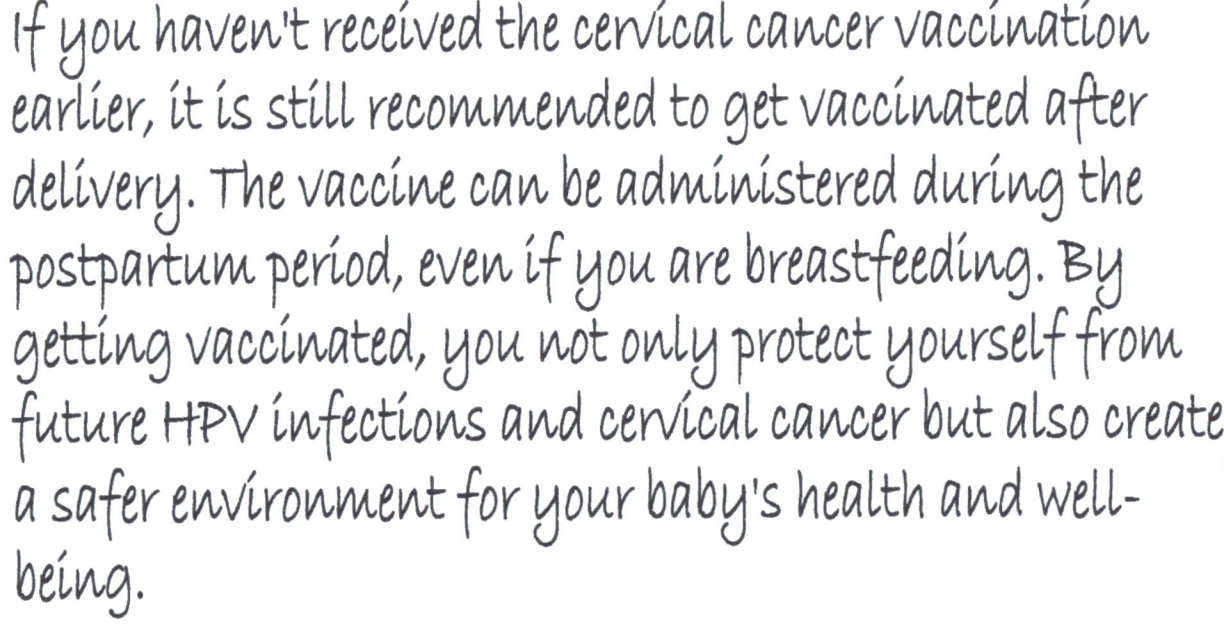

CONCLUSION

Cervical cancer vaccination plays a crucial role in preventing cervical cancer, a disease that affects millions of women worldwide. If you missed the opportunity to get vaccinated earlier, it's never too late to consider getting vaccinated after delivery. By taking this important step, you can safeguard your health and ensure a brighter future, free from the risks and burdens of cervical cancer. Remember to consult with your healthcare provider to discuss your specific circumstances and make an informed decision about cervical cancer vaccination.

Title: Dr. Amrita Saha: Empowering Women through Medicine and Leadership

Introduction:
Dr. Amrita Saha, a dedicated and accomplished gynecologist, is a beacon of hope for women seeking quality healthcare and guidance. With an impressive array of qualifications, extensive experience, and a passion for empowering women, Dr. Saha has made significant contributions to the fields of gynecology and obstetrics. Her journey from a skilled clinician to a compassionate leader has inspired many, leading her to compile her experiences into a scrapbook-style guidebook titled "Mommypedia." This article aims to celebrate Dr. Amrita Saha's remarkable achievements and shed light on her invaluable contributions to women's healthcare.

Education and Specializations:
Dr. Amrita Saha embarked on her medical journey in 2005, graduating with an MBBS degree from the esteemed North Bengal Medical College in Darjeeling. Determined to specialize further, she pursued her MS in Gynecology and Obstetrics from Medical College Kolkata, where she honed her skills and deepened her knowledge in the field.
Driven by her thirst for knowledge, Dr. Saha has also undertaken numerous specialized courses and fellowships. She completed a Master's Course in Cosmetic Gynecology, an Advance Fellowship in Infertility, and a Fellowship in Critical Care Obstetrics. These additional qualifications have not only expanded her expertise but have also allowed her to provide comprehensive care to her patients.

Leadership and Administration:
Dr. Saha's passion for making a difference in healthcare led her to venture into hospital administration. For eight years, she served as the administrator of Fortune Hospital, a prestigious 161-bedded NABH-accredited facility in Kanpur. Her leadership skills and dedication earned her the esteemed recognition of the Best Female Entrepreneur Award.
Throughout her tenure, Dr. Saha ensured the delivery of high-quality healthcare services, prioritizing patient safety and satisfaction. Her exceptional management abilities and commitment to excellence contributed to the hospital's reputation as a center of excellence in women's healthcare.

Research and Publications:
Beyond her clinical and administrative responsibilities, Dr. Amrita Saha is a prolific researcher and academician. She has made significant contributions to the medical community through numerous national and international publications. Her research papers and articles have shed light on various aspects of gynecology and obstetrics, expanding the collective knowledge in the field. Dr. Saha's expertise has been sought after, and she has been invited to speak and participate in prestigious conferences such as AICOG, ISOPARB, North Zone Yuva FOGSI, and UPCOG.

Mommypedia: A Scrapbook and Guidebook
Driven by her desire to empower women and share her wealth of knowledge, Dr. Saha is currently working on a unique project titled "Mommypedia." This scrapbook guidebook aims to provide expecting and new mothers with comprehensive information and guidance on various aspects of pregnancy, childbirth, and postnatal care. Drawing from her vast experience as a gynecologist, Dr. Saha's book promises to be an invaluable resource for women navigating the journey of motherhood.

Conclusion:
Dr. Amrita Saha's journey from a skilled gynecologist to a compassionate leader and author is truly inspiring. Her commitment to providing exceptional healthcare, her extensive qualifications, and her dedication to empowering women have made her a trusted figure in the field. Through her scrapbook and guidebook, "Mommypedia," Dr. Saha continues to make a lasting impact on the lives of countless women. Her legacy serves as a testament to the transformative power of medicine and the strength of determined individuals striving to improve the world around them.

www.ingramcontent.com/pod-product-compliance
Lightning Source LLC
LaVergne TN
LVHW070408070526
838199LV00038B/719